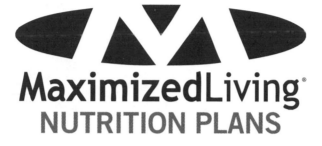

MaximizedLiving®
NUTRITION PLANS

THE SOLUTION TO THE DANGERS OF MODERN NUTRITION
Real nutrition for a healthy body and mind
Discover the scientific solution for weight loss
Lose weight, even if nothing else has worked
Build a thriving family
Balance and regulate your hormones through diet
Stop, prevent, and even reverse diet-related chronic disease

By Dr. B.J. Hardick, Kimberly Roberto, and *New York Times* Best-Selling Author Dr. Ben Lerner

Maximized Living®
Celebration, Florida

Maximized Living®
1170 Celebration Blvd., Suite 100B
Celebration, FL 34747

Maximized Living Nutrition Plans

$24.98
ISBN 978-0-578-03327-3
52498

9 780578 033273

For more information about Maximized Living® or to obtain additional copies of Maximized Living Nutrition Plans, contact Maximized Living® at 321-939-3060 or info@maximizedliving.com.

Revised: March 2015

Table of Contents

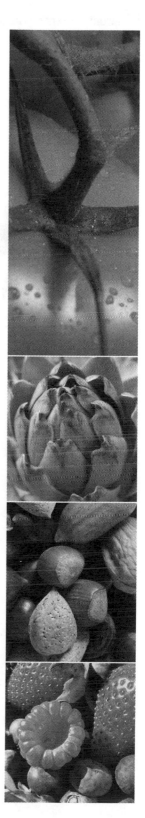

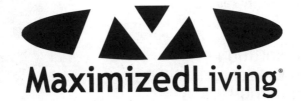

Special Thanks to Contributors:

Dr. Joel Bohemier
Lin Hardick
Evelyn Kooistra
Traci Mahan
Dr. Adam Meade
Dr. Marty Nalda
Kari Penner
Dr. Fred Roberto
Tal Thompson

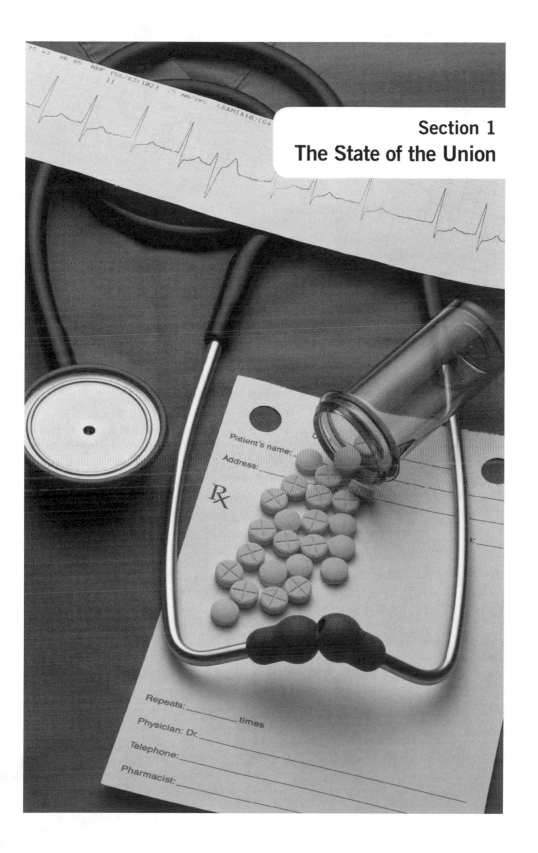

Section 1
The State of the Union

Foreword

By Dr. Ben Lerner, *New York Times* Best-Selling Author, U.S. Olympic and World Team Doctor, Chairman of the USA Wrestling Wellness Advisory Council, Chairman of Global Wellness for the Billion Soul Initiative, and Co-founder of Maximized Living.

Saving the Planet through Nutrition and Maximized Living

Welcome to perhaps the most life-changing tool you'll ever utilize. While that may seem like a "promise too-good-to-be-true," we can assure you that due to the science, the value of the information, the assistance-support materials, and the hundreds of doctors who are trained to help you — we're prepared to deliver on that promise.

My wife, Dr. Sheri Lerner, and I both graduated nearly twenty years ago with bachelor's degrees in nutrition, in addition to our other degrees. Since then, we've carefully tracked the progression of the science of nutrition and have applied these principles with our patients, several U.S. World and Olympic teams, numerous professional sports teams, and through hundreds of chiropractic clinics worldwide. Because of the training, certification, and size of our network, I doubt a more clinically tested series of programs and recommendations exists in the world.

We've seen firsthand the challenges people encounter when trying to eat well. Not only is it difficult to find a plan that is easy to follow and successful, but it can be overwhelming to navigate through all the different and sometimes conflicting information that is available. As a result, conditions related to nutrition and other critical areas of lifestyle are causing adults and children to become sicker than ever. Fortunately, with this book and our help, you'll find that this suffering is unnecessary, reversible, and best of all — preventable.

State of the Union

The United States spends an astounding $2.3 trillion annually on healthcare — radically more than any other country spends. This is 4.3 times the amount spent on military defense. Yet, the World Health Organization ranks U.S. healthcare only 37th among organized nations, about even with Serbia. Canada ranks 30th. Shockingly, North American countries spend twice as much per capita on healthcare as European countries, yet we are twice as sick with chronic disease. Currently, 75 percent of healthcare costs are accounted for by chronic diseases, such as heart disease, diabetes, prostate cancer, breast cancer, and obesity. (Keehan, et al, Health Affairs.)

What these five diseases and conditions have in common is that they are largely preventable and even reversible by changes in lifestyle and bodily function. In a statement to the U.S. Senate Health Committee, Dr. Dean Ornish stated: "Studies have shown that changing lifestyle could prevent at least 90 percent of all heart disease. Thus, the disease that accounts for more premature deaths and costs Americans more than any other illness is almost completely preventable, and even reversible, simply by changing lifestyle." (Harkin, examiner.com)

While most people and many doctors still do not acknowledge this fact, the truth is poor diet and lifestyle are primary killers. Gone are the days when you could blame poor genetics and bad luck for your illness or conditions. You also can no longer believe that the only solutions to health problems are medical doctors, drugs, and surgery. Countless studies expose the reality that the most common deadly conditions, although caused by unhealthy living, can be reversed by implementing better lifestyle choices.

The sudden increase in obese children, and the concern over the catastrophic consequences this will have for the future, should be a huge wake-up call for all of us. Chronic conditions, such as heart disease, cancer, and diabetes, previously seen only in adults, are now becoming prevalent in young adults and children. One in every four American children is seriously overweight or at risk of becoming overweight. In the United States, 30 percent of boys and 40 percent of girls are at risk for developing type 2 diabetes – an obesity related condition – sometime in their lives. In the 1990s, type 2 diabetes accounted for up to 45 percent of all new pediatric cases of diabetes, compared to fewer than 4 percent before the 1990s. Experts now say that we're looking at the first generation of children who will experience a shorter life expectancy than their parents. (Bibbins-Domingo, *New England Journal of Medicine.*)

At this point in our culture, the focus of the solution has been how to get people more health insurance – or how to get the government to pay for it. Yet, it makes absolutely no sense to simply figure out how to better pay the bills. We have to figure out how to stop getting sick in the first place.

While endless promises are made by books, Web sites, infomercials, drugs, and doctors of all kinds, the truth is we're just getting sicker, fatter, and more miserable. Something is obviously missing from the healthcare equation. Based on statistics on prescription-drug use and disease, it's been estimated that only one in a thousand people by the age of sixty are actually in any decent level of health and not taking medication for chronic illness. We want you to be one more person living a Maximized Life.

To Get Started, Ask Yourself:

- When was the last time you were able to wake up in the morning energized and refreshed without the use of coffee or other stimulants?

- What would it be like to feel good all of the time?

- Can you imagine looking your best every day?

The body was actually designed to do these things and do them for a long time. You only need to watch Willard Scott on the *Today Show* with his Smuckers® segment to see that there are people hitting 100 every day. These are your neighbors, with your genetics, and not some random people living on a mountaintop in the Far East.

This book will reveal the secrets you need to know in the area of nutrition. Let me start by uncomplicating the foundations of the science of nutrition, because they actually are quite easy to understand. You learned about them as early as a junior high history class.

- We all remember what happened when the sailors crossed the ocean without lemons and developed vitamin C deficiency – scurvy.

- Older generations remember what happens when children didn't have access to vitamin D — rickets.

- Most of us have seen the commercials showing children throughout Africa who are starving to death yet have protruding bellies. The condition is called kwashiorkor, a disease of protein deficiency.

Therefore, it's simple: If your diet lacks certain key nutrients, it's exposed to the possibility of severe and debilitating disease that, if not corrected, can lead to death.

We also know what happens to people whose food and/or water supply expose them to harm.

I remember an eighth-grade lesson on "Mad-hatters Disease" in which hatters began to lose their minds and go "mad" because the material they were handling, namely fur and felt, had been treated with mercury. This is not too different from today when water and food sources regularly become contaminated with germs and toxins. These poisons enter our systems and make us physically or mentally ill.

Similarly, it has become evident that those who eat too much sugar, bad fats, and fried foods find themselves obese, with a far higher incidence of disease and earlier death than their healthier-eating counterparts.

<u>So, the foundations of nutrition are not too hard to understand:</u> Diet deficiency in what you do need, and/or overindulgence in what you do not, leads to illness, madness, (depression, sleeplessness, and anxiety), big bellies, buns, and thighs.

Despite these easy-to-understand principles, many people and their doctors still stand in denial and continue to keep the fast-food restaurants and refined-food industries booming, which in turn keeps drug companies and Big and Tall stores profiting, as well.

Now that you know the simple, easy-to-comprehend foundations of nutrition, you will understand why what we've been doing for the last two decades has been so successful.

When we address the issue of obesity, along with the ever-increasing challenges of pain, depression, and disease, we don't "treat" these problems like conventional medicine or common nutrition practices do.

There was a time, when the only condition associated with food was "tight pants" — being overweight or fat. Over time, that condition no longer was blamed on unhealthy eating. Instead, people blamed "bad glands" or "poor genetics." However, now we know everything from heart disease and cancer to depression and zits is connected to what we eat.

For example, there was a British prison study done at *Aylesbury* jail that showed that when the young male inmates were fed certain critical vitamins and essential fatty acids, the number of violent offenses committed in the prison fell by 37 per cent. *(Sydney Morning Herald)*

This is not a unique trial. A multitude of literature exists confirming the powerful impact certain nutrients, particularly omega-3 fats, have on mental and physical health. What's more important than the results, however, is the reason behind the result.

Like sailors with scurvy, or African children with kwashiorkor, if your diet is deficient, there's an unpleasant consequence. If you give the sailors a lime, or one of the starving children a piece of salmon, the disease — if caught in time — will disappear completely. Does this mean you "treated" the disease with fruit and fish? No. You simply provided the proper nutrients required by your body for good health

So, while studies show that "omega-3s are beneficial for treating depression," or some expert says that "vitamin C is good for treating a cold," what's really happening is that there has been a deficiency or imbalance in these nutrients all along that led to a symptom or "disease."

The key terms here are:

1. Deficiency and 2. Imbalance.

   1. Deficiency comes largely from replacing whole foods and good choices with processed bad ones. Deficiency also is the result of the body's inability to actually digest the nutrients even if you are ingesting them.

   2. Imbalance comes from deficiency—too much of one type of nutrient without enough of another to balance it. But imbalance also comes from modern methods of food production. For example, the importance in supplementing with an essential fatty acid, such as omega-3, is not just digesting enough of it but getting the right balance of omega-3s to omega-6s.

Imbalances also come from modern methods of food production. If cows are raised eating their normal diet of grass, the meat produced will have the right balance of omega-3 to omega-6 fats. However, if cows are fed grain, the omega-3 content is lost. The key with omega-3 is not just digesting enough of it, but getting the right ratio of omega-3s to omega-6s. If there are too many 6s and not enough 3s, you'll develop many of the problems victims of modern food production face today — inflammation, weight gain, depression, and disease.

Dr. Joseph Hibbeln, psychiatrist and physician, has found that if you measure omega-3 and omega-6 in people with mood disorders, omega-3 is often low while omega-6 is increased. Dr. Hibbeln, responsible for a study on mood and aggression in the United States, thinks that today's commercial diets very well may be "changing the very architecture and functioning of the brain." (Gupta, CNN)

As the United States and the ever-growing populations adopting our diets shift from foods high in omega-3s to diets rich in soy, corn, sunflower, and other commercial oils used in packaged and fast foods, which are high in omega-6, we're creating a painful and deadly imbalance. On the other hand, with so many people wolfing down omega-3s today, some people have an imbalance the other way, which leads to its own kind of health problems. The key is getting it right. And when we get it right, imagine what this will mean for children and adults around the world.

In this book, you will see a sane, scientifically supported way of getting back to eating the way you were intended to eat, so that you avoid deficiency and create the balance you need. My good friends and nutrition experts, Dr. B.J. Hardick and Kimberly Roberto, have helped create an incredible resource for families and individuals of any age and from any walk of life.

We're going to show you how to have it all: good looks and great health. We want you alive, living your potential, looking great, fulfilling a purpose, and perhaps most importantly, being a role model of good health for your family and future generations. Together, we'll save the planet.

Chapter 1

What Happened?

Sugar

Sugar: The "Staple Food" of the Standard North American Diet

If you were alive in the 1980s, you may recall the statistic, "every can of Coke® has 9 teaspoons of sugar." Sadly, twenty years later, that number is now 13 teaspoons. Sugar content not only has been on the rise in soda but in most of today's packaged foods, which make up the bulk of the Standard North American Diet.

John Robbins, the biological heir to the Baskin-Robbins® ice cream fortune, turned down the opportunity to take over his family enterprise when he learned what the Standard North American Diet was doing to people. He writes in his book, *Healthy at 100*, that as of 2006:

"The average American consumes 53 teaspoons of sugar per day."

That number might seem impossible. It is the equivalent of a five-pound bag of sugar being consumed by every man, woman, and child every ten days. A major source of caloric intake in North Americans has become soda, which is packed with sugar. In fact, many of the lemon-lime drinks contain more sugar per serving than the traditional cola drinks. The average American now consumes 55 gallons of soda per year. Soda makes up 10 percent-15 percent of teenage girls' caloric intake. Families switching to juice aren't doing their children any favors either. American children between the ages of six and eleven each consume approximately 19 gallons of juice per year — and each serving of juice, on average, contains more sugar than a serving of soda.

If you look in your pantry, you may be surprised to find sugar added to your pasta sauce, lunch meats, canned soups, condiments, and even table salt. For that reason, it doesn't take much to reach your 53 teaspoons per day. Robbins makes the important point in *Healthy at 100* that in countries where whole cultures of people live to reach 100 in great health, they consume no refined sugar whatsoever.

Unfortunately, Robbins' numbers may be an underestimate. Although "white foods" (white bread, white rice, and white pasta), may not list many grams of sugar on their labels, the moment the food touches the digestive enzymes in saliva, they break down into simple sugar within seconds. And that contributes to overall sugar consumption. Starting with refined flour, these white foods make up the base of the traditional food pyramid. And although governments recommend that we consume more whole grains on a regular basis, even the "whole," healthy foods are often disguised. "Whole wheat" bread in the grocery store typically has "whole wheat" added to white flour, which in its simplest form is sugar. *(Robbins, Healthy at 100.)*

What is the deal with sugar?

Sugar is cheap and addictive. These two qualities make it manufacturers' perfect additive to nearly every boxed food in today's grocery store. You will keep coming back for more "tasty" food, and you will justify the expense by how little it costs. Unfortunately, you'll be consuming the number one food risk factor for diabetes, heart disease, and cancer.

While you may be trying to do your best by switching to "natural" and "organic" brands, don't be fooled. Organic sugar, maple syrup, honey, and cane juice, while less processed than white sugar, have the same negative impact on your body. The emphasis should be on the word "sugar," not the word "organic." While organic manufacturers must meet guide-lines to label their foods organic, those guidelines are not endorsed by Maximized Living. Organic sugar is still sugar.

If you've attempted to eliminate white flour from your diet, and have moved strictly to whole grains, think again. You may be shocked to see refined flour appear on your labels, in addition to a whole host of other additives. If you have done very well and selected items that contain only "100 percent whole grains," it is only a matter of seconds before your body breaks down the fiber, germ, and bran of the grain, leaving the endosperm, the sugar of the plant, to wreak havoc on your body.

Historically, we consumed sugar derived from the bush known as sugar cane. However, sugar cane grew in limited quantities on North American soil, and a more economical source of sugar was soon derived from the cornfields of the Midwest: high-fructose corn syrup. More potent than white sugar, high-fructose corn syrup is now used in soda — explaining why the average can of Coke® has 13 teaspoons of sugar, instead of "only" 9. (Robbins, *Healthy at 100.)* Corn is now the number one source of sugar products used in America, specifically in its derivatives, which include corn syrup, high-fructose corn syrup, corn oil, corn meal, corn starch, dextrose, xanthan gum, and maltodextrin. Wheat is the number one North American source of refined flour, which may not be listed as sugar on the label, but nonetheless will cause the same problems.

So, why is there so much talk about the consumption of sugar? After all, we've traditionally been taught that it is excess fat that causes heart disease and obesity, while sugar provides energy and is acceptable in moderation. In truth, the number one dietary cause of heart disease and the obesity epidemic is the amount of carbohydrates we consume.

Obesity

When sugar enters the body, it is broken down into its simplest form for appropriate use. The sugar is then moved into the bloodstream for transport. The body can function in a state of health — homeostasis — and optimal performance when there are approximately 1-2 teaspoons of sugar in the bloodstream. In greater quantities, your body faces the risk of coma, or even death. Therefore, when faced with excess sugar, as it is daily in North Americans, the body uses insulin to move the sugar out of the blood and into the cells so that it can be used for energy. In the average North American, because there is so much sugar consumed and available in the body, not all of it can be used as energy. Therefore, the body must do something with the excess sugar once in the cells. The body's solution: **store the excess sugar as fat.**

Type 2 Diabetes

The need for your body to move sugar into the cells for energy, rather than leave it in the bloodstream, requires the hormone insulin to move sugar across the cell membrane. Insulin, produced by the pancreas, binds to insulin receptors on the cell membrane to bring sugar into the cells to be converted into energy. While this system is effective to a point, the constant bombardment of sugar and elevation of insulin eventually causes the insulin receptors to burn out. The result is elevated blood sugar, in other words: diabetes. The long-term complications of diabetes include vision damage, kidney dysfunction, heart disease, neurological paresthesia in the body, and poor healing of wounds, which can lead to amputation of limbs.

The good news is that our Advanced Plan (page 49) is specifically designed to reverse the damage done by years of sugar consumption, to assist type-2 diabetics restore normal body chemistry, and to regenerate the insulin receptors previously destroyed.

Cancer

In 1931, German Professor Otto Warburg received the Nobel Prize in Physiology or Medicine for his studies showing that cancer cells and tumors generate energy by glycolysis, the non-oxidative breakdown of glucose in the absence of oxygen. Fundamentally, Dr. Warburg hypothesized that cancer cells use sugar as their main source of energy, in contrast with healthy cells, which use oxygen.

When insulin levels become high, in response to high blood sugar, the liver releases IGF-1 (Insulin-like Growth Factor), which causes the cells of the body to grow in the presence of food. Cancer cells have eight times the number of receptors of IGF-1 than do healthy cells of the body and therefore utilize sugar as their primary fuel. Furthermore, IGF-1 has an estrogen-like action, making it very dangerous in hormone-responsive cancers, such as breast cancer. IGF-1 also promotes the formation of blood vessels in tumors, allowing cancers to grow and spread.

Not only does sugar feed cancerous cells, it also impedes the function of the immune system, which would otherwise identify and destroy potentially mutated and harmful cells.

Remember, cancer is not caught like a cold. We all have 100 to 10,000 cancer cells in our body at any moment in time. The way to prevent cancer cells from spreading is to maintain a strong immune system and not fuel them with their number one food choice: sugar.

"Cancer, above all other diseases, has countless secondary causes. But, even for cancer, there is only one prime cause. Summarized in a few words, the prime cause of cancer is the replacement of the respiration of oxygen in normal body cells by a fermentation of sugar." ~ Dr. Otto Warburg

Top 10 Reasons to Avoid Sugar and Refined Grains

1. **Sugar is the primary dietary cause of the obesity epidemic.**
   Fat doesn't make you fat. But sugar that turns into fat will.

2. **Sugar causes hormonal and metabolic imbalance.**
   Swinging insulin and cortisol levels in the body, which decrease then increase blood sugar, not only cause your system to crash but set up a cascade of abnormal hormone functions that lead to premature aging and illness.

3. **Sugar is your fast track to diabetes.**
   On the Standard North American Diet, it is only a matter of time before insulin receptors burn out, unable to handle the onslaught of sugar.

4. **Sugar increases the acidity of the body.**
   All disease thrives in acidic environments.

5. **Sugar causes inflammation.**
   Inflammatory enzymes are elevated on higher-sugar diets. Inflammation is at the heart of 98 percent of disease.

6. **Sugar is the primary reason for high cholesterol.**
   Your body's innate healing system, which uses cholesterol, goes into high gear when the body is traumatized at the cellular level by high sugar, insulin, and inflammation. The solution to high cholesterol is not to lower it forcefully but to remove the interference in the body causing it to rise in the first place.

7. **Sugar leads to heart disease.**
   Elevated inflammation in the arteries increases the risk of high blood pressure, hemorrhage, stroke, and heart attacks.

8. **Sugar is an anti-nutrient.**
   Your body's expenditure to manage sugar is greater than the energy it gains from it. If you think you are better off eating a chocolate bar, or piece of white bread, than going hungry — think again.

9. **Sugar is a known toxin.**
   Like all toxins, your body is constantly trying to eliminate it from the bloodstream. You can assist your body by not giving it more sugar to handle.

10. **Sugar promotes cancer.**
    Feeding cancer cells their primary fuel is like pouring gas on a fire.

(Warburg, *The Prime Cause and Prevention of Cancer.)*

While medical theorists and pharmaceutical companies have proposed many other causes of cancer since Dr. Warburg's research, his principle that cancer cells switch to glycolysis remains widely accepted today and continues to be utilized in the development of cancer drugs. However, wouldn't it make better sense to eliminate the cause of the problem, rather than develop medications to combat the symptoms?

The Low-Fat / High-Obesity Diet

For more than thirty years, the low-fat diet has been promoted in the Western world as the means to healthy arteries and a slim figure. This message has propelled 15,000 low-fat products onto the shelves of North American supermarkets. Clearly, the message to avoid fat in foods has become deeply embedded in the minds of North Americans.

While we now have more low-fat foods and low-fat diets compared with any other part of the world, we also have the highest rate of obesity — and this trend has come as a direct result of our obsession with low-fat foods. Since the 1970s, North Americans' dietary fat consumption has dropped from 40 percent to 34 percent while the rate of obesity has increased from 14 percent to 22 percent. (Burne, *Health: The Myth of the Low-Fat Diet*)

The American Heart Association follows these rules for a 2,000-calorie-per day, low-fat diet:

• 6-8 servings of grains, with at least half from whole grains
• 4-5 servings of raw or cooked vegetables
• 4-5 servings of fruit
• 2-3 servings of non-fat or low-fat dairy products
• 6 ounces of lean protein
• 2 servings of fat and oils
• 2-3 servings of nuts, seeds, or legumes per week
• 5 servings of sweets/sugar per week

When this diet is analyzed by carbohydrate, protein, and fat content, then compared with caloric content, it calculates to:

• 68 percent carbohydrate
• 12 percent protein
• 20 percent fat

By any standard, the low-fat diet is also a high-carbohydrate diet, which we now know has a negative impact on blood sugar, insulin metabolism, cancer, and obesity. Its effect on heart disease, which affects 50 percent of Americans, is frightening.

The Lipid Hypothesis

One of the goals of the low-fat diet is to lower cholesterol, which traditionally has been thought to be the culprit behind heart disease. Consumption of saturated fat in particular, we are told, must be substantially lowered on the low-fat diet for the purpose of lowering cholesterol. If diet alone doesn't work, doctors will prescribe powerful statin drugs to forcefully lower one's cholesterol levels. Some physicians will prescribe cholesterol-lowering medications in conjunction with their patients' diet and exercise, asserting that cholesterol levels must be lowered at any cost. (Carey, *Business Week*)

Unfortunately, while the government and most doctors endorse the low-fat, low-saturated fat, and low-cholesterol diets, (or regime of cholesterol-lowering medications), the evidence to support the "lipid hypothesis" that implies elevated fat and cholesterol in the blood causes heart disease is questionable at best.

No randomized research study has ever been able to link a low-fat diet and lower cholesterol to a lower risk of coronary heart disease. In fact, according to published research:

- More people have heart attacks with normal cholesterol than with elevated cholesterol.
- There is a higher death rate among people with low cholesterol than with high cholesterol. (Wannamethee, et al, *British Medical Journal, et al.*)

During the past two generations of North Americans living the low-fat lifestyle, mortality rates from coronary heart disease, cancer, and diabetes have actually been rising. (Ford, et al, *Coronary Heart Disease Mortality Among Young Adults in the U.S. From 1980 Through 2002: Concealed Leveling of Mortality Rates, et al.*) Fortunately, not all countries are following our lead, such as the following:

France
In France, the levels of saturated fat intake are much higher than they are in the United States, yet the French and Spanish have much lower rates of death from cardiovascular disease. (Ferrieres, *The French Paradox: Lessons for Other Countries.*)

The French eat four times more butter and 60 percent more cheese than Americans.

Although the French eat slightly more fat overall, they actually eat a great deal more saturated fat than Americans, who have exchanged their consumption of saturated fat for unsaturated fats such as vegetable oils, canola oil, and soybean oil.

How are the French doing? According to data from the British Heart foundation, in 1999, rates of death from coronary heart disease among males ages 35–74 was nearly 30 percent less in France than it was in America. (Sekikawa, *Why Heart Disease Mortality Is Low in France*)

Spain
A 1995 study in the *American Journal of Clinical Nutrition* reviewed trends in deaths from coronary heart disease and stroke in Spain from 1966-1990, with respect to dietary changes.

The study found that since 1976, there had been a **decrease** in cardiovascular-disease deaths in both men and women in Spain. During the same period that coronary heart disease and stroke death rates fell, the national intake of meat, dairy products, and fish increased in Spain. Meanwhile, the intake of sugar, carbohydrates, and olive oil, which is low in saturated fat, decreased. If saturated fat was the cause of heart disease, why did the death rate go down?

East Africa

A study of the Masai tribes in Kenya, East Africa, shows that their diet consists of full-fat milk and cream, large amounts of beef, and even the blood of their cattle during the dry season. The Masai men consume almost a pound of saturated fat on a daily basis.

Examinations of the Masai by Western physicians revealed some interesting findings: The Masai's blood cholesterol levels were extremely low. Autopsies of deceased Masai have found virtually no evidence of arterial plaque. (Amin, et al, *The Last of the Masai*, 87.)

These findings are in direct contradiction to our belief that eating saturated fat causes high cholesterol levels and hardening of the arteries.

"The hypothesis has been repeatedly shown to be wrong; and yet, for complicated reasons of pride, profit, and prejudice, the hypothesis continues to be exploited by scientists, fund-raising enterprises, food companies and even governmental agencies. The public is being deceived by the greatest health scam of the century." ~ George Mann, Sc.D., M.D., former co-director, The Framingham Study (Mann, *New England Journal of Medicine*)

Healthy Fat vs. Damaged Fat

The reporting of fats in the media has caused most of us to think that all fat is bad. While it's true that some fats are dangerous for your health, it's inaccurate to lump all fats together. The truth is not all fats are bad; some are quite beneficial.

Generally speaking, the North American studies, which linked fat with disease, have evaluated the impact of unhealthy or damaged fats on the body — and overlooked the incredible benefits of healthy fats. Instead of comparing healthy fats with damaged fats, we have erroneously assumed that all fats are the enemy. The concept of "low fat" has been grossly simplified to include both healthy and damaged fats. This has led the studies to incorrectly conclude that eating a diet high in healthy fats is harmful.

Healthy Fats include olive oil, avocados, nuts, seeds, coconuts, and the fats that come from naturally-raised animals, including wild fish and grass-fed beef.

Healthy Fats provide your body with the nutrients it needs to build cell membranes, absorb vitamins, cushion vital organs, protect you from extreme temperatures, build hormones, lower inflammation, and make up 70 percent of your brain tissue.

Damaged Fats are fats that are altered in the process of extracting them from their sources, as they are assimilated in your body, or during the manufacturing process, as in the case of hydrogenated oils (trans fats).

Damaged Fats have no place in your diet. Since your body cannot recognize or metabolize these fats, they naturally contribute to weight gain by clinging to cell membranes and preventing cellular detoxification. Beyond the concern of weight loss, these damaged fats also adhere to arterial walls, cause inflammation and damage, and contribute to heart attacks and stroke. The natural rise in cholesterol, in response to the damage caused by such fats, is the body's attempt to heal itself. Unfortunately, we've been led to believe that taking medications to forcefully lower the number of "healing agents" in the body will address the true cause of the problem — when clearly, it won't.

Damaged Fats include:

Trans fats (hydrogenated oils) — The world is waking up to the realization that altering foods is harmful to consumers. Hydrogen, forced into otherwise non-hydrogenated oils, causes these fats to become more stable at room temperature, thereby extending the shelf life of candy bars and packaged foods. However, this process also changes the composition of fats from a state that can be recognized by your body to one that cannot be recognized and as a result may have deadly consequences.

Even our governing bodies are advising people to stay away from trans fats. Restaurants in major American cities have made pacts to stop using them. However, trans fats are not banned completely from the manufacturing process and often remain hidden in today's foods. For example, if the trans fat content <u>per serving</u> is less than 500 milligrams, foods may be deceivingly labeled as "trans-fat free." Manufacturers have simply reduced their serving size to meet this advertising standard. Even the manufacturers would agree that according to their own definition of "serving size," once you've eaten your eighth potato chip, your snack is no longer "trans-fat free."

Vegetable oil is processed by chemical extraction using solvent extracts that will produce quick, cheap, and high yields of oil to be used in foods. Vegetable oil's primary uses include adding texture and flavor to foods. Vegetable oils prevent the "sticking-together" of other ingredients. In the case of shortening, it gives pastries that crumbly texture. The flavors of vegetable oils are carried well, since many of the flavors present in chemicals are soluble in the oil. Vegetable oils are found in nearly every packaged food and salad dressing in the grocery store. They include soybean oil, corn oil, safflower oil, cottonseed oil, canola oil, and others simply labeled as "vegetable oil."

Vegetables aren't unhealthy. But their oils become harmful when they are unnaturally extracted from their sources. Vegetable oil belongs in the vegetable, not in your box of crackers or your frying pan.

There are two primary health hazards associated with vegetable oils. First, these fats are typically high in omega-6 fats, rather than omega-3 fats for which most Americans are severely deficient if they are eating the Standard North American Diet. The overabundance of omega-6 fats in our diets has disrupted the natural and ideal ratio of 4:1 omega-6 to omega-3 fats in our bodies. This imbalance has been associated with elevated inflammation and obstructed blood circulation. It is vital to maintain a 4:1 ratio of omega-6 to omega-3 fats in the diet. While most North Americans are already well above the 4:1 ratio, often 20:1 or even 50:1, additional vegetable oil in the diet creates further problems.

Beyond the problems associated with a poor ratio of omega-6 and omega-3 fats are the problems associated with rancidification, which is the decomposition of fats, by exposure to air, heat, or light, causing oils to oxidize and form free radicals. The splitting of fatty acid chains away from their molecular backbones allows the free fatty acids to undergo further oxidation. Free radicals are unquestionably related to cancer. Further, chemical breakdown destroys the nutrients needed by your body, and will create a compound that is hazardous to your health.

Rancidification may occur in the manufacturing plant, in the bottle, or in your body — but it is not required by law to be reported on the food label. While we've traditionally been told to stay away from saturated fat, science indicates that we should take an opposite approach. In fact, saturated fats are least likely to be affected by oxidation because they are very stable and have a high degree of resistance. Monounsaturated fats like olive oil are somewhat vulnerable to oxidation, since they have one pair of missing hydrogen atoms. Vegetable oils are polyunsaturated, as they are missing several pairs of hydrogen atoms, and are therefore highly unstable and the most susceptible.

Polyunsaturated vegetable oils are so vulnerable to becoming rancid that even at room temperature and in subdued light, oxidation occurs inside the bottle. The oils have been refined and deodorized so that you can't smell or taste the chemical decomposition of the oils — but you can be certain that all polyunsaturated vegetable oils sold at grocery stores have become rancid to some degree even before you bring them home. And what has not become rancid in the box or bottle will become rancid in your body once ingested.

Canola oil needs special attention. This oil does not occur in nature. In fact, there is no such thing as a canola plant growing anywhere on our planet. Canola oil is a genetic manipulation of rapeseed oil, altered to reduce its levels of toxic erucic acid. Originally called "Lear" oil, standing for "Low Erucic Acid Rapeseed" oil, the name was changed to the more consumer-friendly "Canola" oil, meaning "Canadian Oil Low Acid."

Canola oil is often touted as one of the healthiest oils because of its low saturated fat content, which we now know is nothing to boast of, and its similarity to olive oil in terms of its monounsaturated content. However, not only is canola oil manmade, but during the manufacturing process the healthy omega-3 fats are denatured making it unrecognizable and unusable by the body. Furthermore, the denaturing process creates a horrible odor, which is removed by additional heating of the oil at 300°F. Since vegetable oils are not stable when heated, this process further denatures the omega-3's fats and causes rancidity.

Butter vs. Margarine

Margarine, a trans fat, was developed and introduced to the world markets in an effort to shift people away from eating butter, a saturated fat. Not surprisingly, heart disease escalated in the years when margarine consumption increased 300 percent, and the consumption of butter was cut in half. Even so, many nutritionists and doctors still recommend the use of margarine as a heart-friendly option.

Butter, consumed by cultures for hundreds of years without any elevated risk of heart disease, contains arachidonic acid and conjugated linoleic acid, vital for brain function and fat metabolism. Its apparent demise is strictly a result of the low-fat movement. But recently, butter has been making a comeback.

While newer margarines and similar "spreads" are made with non-hydrogenated oils, they are in fact polyunsaturated, rancid vegetable oils that are harmful to the human body.

Hormones and Fat Metabolism

While the damaged fats are clearly unhealthy at the cellular level, healthy fats are your body's preferred source of energy. Per gram of consumption, healthy fats provide twice the energy of protein or carbohydrates. This excess of calories will only turn into body fat if your body doesn't know how to use it. Fat metabolism is not controlled by your caloric intake, but by your hormones.

Myth: Fat makes you fat.
Truth: The inability to burn fat is what makes you fat.

While 25 percent to 30 percent of North Americans are clinically obese, less than 10 percent of the French are obese by the same standards.

Fat does not make you fat. A 2009 study by the American College of Cardiology examined and tested 645 obese and overweight patients using high- and low-fat diets. Despite the differences in protein, fat and carbohydrate intake, there was **no change** in waist circumference between each group. This means that the "low-fat group" didn't get any smaller over the course of the study. The mean weight loss for the high-fat diet group in this study was 7.3 pounds. The mean weight loss for the low-fat group was 7.3 pounds. — a difference of zero pounds. (Bavry, *The American College of Cardiology*)

Leptin

Your body's ability or inability to burn fat is under the ultimate control of leptin, "the fat-burning hormone" discovered in 1994.

Leptin is a hormone produced by your fat cells and delivered to the brain's hypothalamus to regulate fat burning, hunger, cravings, and the sense of being "full." Slightly increased leptin, released from the fat cells and detected in the brain, causes the body to burn fat for energy.

Leptin is described as your body's "gas gauge" for determining when to eat and "stock up" on nutrients — versus when to burn fat for energy in the absence of food. During hunter-gatherer times, leptin played a vital role for survival, because humans would go for days without eating. In modern times, leptin is no longer the survival mechanism; and unfortunately for many, it has become the enemy.

Innately, the amount of leptin produced in the body is proportional to the amount of body fat a person has. Leptin provides the necessary signal to the brain to perceive how much energy the body has in its reserves to be used during times of starvation, which hardly exists in modern times.

In the last century, fewer North Americans have been faced with a deficiency of food. The vast majority of North Americans get three meals plus several snacks — often more food than is needed for survival. This overabundance of food is largely comprised of empty calories, chemical toxins, and depleted nutrients preventing the body from ever becoming satisfied and actually causing a "starvation" for nutrients.

The body gets "full" from nutrients — not calories.

In hunter-gatherer times, a lack of nutrients would equate to a lack of food. Because fat would be used for energy during any absence of food, leptin levels would automatically drop, signaling the body to slow down the metabolism while on the search for food.

However, in modern times, due to the overabundance and constant snacking of food, the brain never "hears" decreased leptin but instead hears a constant elevation of leptin. As a result, there is no slowing down of the metabolism since the closest meal is typically just one fast-food restaurant away. Whereas slightly elevated leptin would promote fat burning, North American levels of leptin, often two to five times higher than normally elevated levels, actually cause the leptin receptors at the hypothalamus to burn out. Because the brain is no longer capable of detecting increased leptin in the blood, it errone-ously begins to sense a deficiency of leptin and will cause the body to crave more food to impede starvation. This broken barometer in the brain now causes the person to constantly feel hungry, never burn fat as its primary fuel for energy, and continually seek sugar as an immediate source of fulfillment.

Leptin Resistance, also known as **Weight-Loss Resistance**, is the syndrome caused by increased leptin not detected by the brain, due to the burning out of leptin receptors at the hypothalamus.

In addition to the Standard North American Diet causing constantly elevated leptin and leptin resistance, other factors in our diets and lifestyle contribute to this syndrome:

- **Toxicity** - Fat-soluble toxins present in food and the environment, and ingested in our bodies, eventually will find their way into our fat cells causing an unregu-lated release of leptin, which will burn out the brain's leptin receptors.

- **Inflammation** - Toxins in the system create an inflammatory response within our body's cells, mediated by cytokines, which block leptin receptors in the brain.

- **Snacking** — All meals cause some rise in insulin, which causes the body to burn food over fat. This rise in insulin, along with increased consumption of triglyc-erides, prevents the triglyceride levels from being fully cleared from the blood. *Elevated triglycerides — a warning sign that the body does not efficiently use fat for energy — create a negative cascade in which they physically impede the entrance of leptin into the brain.*

Beyond Weight Loss

Whether or not weight is a concern, the imbalance of leptin in the body can cause addi-tional problems:

- In addition to the brain, leptin receptors exist in the heart. Elevated leptin causes an elevation of C-reactive protein, considered to be the most reliable and primary risk factor related to a person's first heart attack or stroke.

- Elevated leptin causes a persistent and unnatural elevation of immune cells and inflammation in the body's fat or adipose tissue, causing damage to the vital organs protected by it.

- Increased inflammation in the body, triggered by leptin, will increase cholesterol and subsequently increase blood pressure, red blood cell adhesiveness, and risk for kidney damage.

Whether or not a person needs to or wants to lose weight, the importance of balancing one's leptin and hormones should be clear to all.

Hormone Repair

Repairing your body's hormones to levels innately experienced during hunter-gatherer times depends on a number of factors related to fat consumption:

To train your body to burn fat, (as opposed to sugar and immediately ingested food), the body needs a good supply of fat in the diet. **Distance yourself from low-fat foods.** When fat is reduced, it is likely to be replaced with refined carbohydrates and sugars. Read your labels (p. 70).

The building block of all hormones is fat. To repair the body's hormones, it needs fat — and a lot of it — in healthy forms.

More critical to the body's chemistry of having the right amount of fat is the consumption of essential fats in the right ratio. The World Health Organization (WHO)-endorsed ideal ratio of omega-6 to omega-3 fats in the body is 4:1. Studies have shown that the treatment of patients with essential fats in the ideal 4:1 ratio yields results not achievable by the administration of any single fatty acid alone. These results include improved brain function, sleep patterns, stress adaptation, and cortisol levels, which influence blood sugar metabolism and weight loss. (Yehuda, *Omega-6/Omega-3 Essential Fatty Acid Ratio: The Scientific Evidence, 37-56.*)

In the 21st century, we are exposed to few examples of healthy physiques compared with our Paleolithic ancestors, or even compared with the generation of our great-grandparents. In an effort to feel and function more in line with our genetic ideals, be sure to follow our meal planning guidelines in Chapter 6 when planning your meals on our Core and Advanced Plans. These rules will help you reach your goals.

Animal Fat — Where to Start

Research continues to show that it is not meat that is the problem — but what we have done to meat. While saturated fat contained in grass-fed meat is critical for brain function, cell function, and the prevention of heart disease, the saturated fat in animals that are fed grains, (not their preferred source of food), becomes denatured and harmful in the human body. **The hundreds of articles linking commercial red meat to cancer and heart disease have consistently studied the impact of grain-fed meats on the human body and overlooked the incredible benefits of animal proteins when consumed in their natural state.**

Cows were designed to roam pastures and eat grass, not grain. When animals are fed grain, their fatty acid ratios soar beyond 20:1, five times greater than the ideal ratio of 4:1. The disruption of chemistry in grain-fed animals is so extreme that these animals would develop acidosis and die at a young age. However, early and timely slaughtering of the animals allows them to enter the food chain while still considered "healthy." Conversely, grass-fed animals live long, healthy lives. These are the animals consumed by the Masai and meat-eating cultures around the world where diseases unique to North America are sparse.

What about Cholesterol?

In spite of the research surrounding the benefits of healthy fats and saturated fats, North Americans have been persuaded by drug ads to fear any elevation of cholesterol. The suggestion that trusted physicians or the American Heart Association may have missed the mark is sometimes difficult to accept.

Cholesterol is necessary to create hormones, to repair cell membranes, to make vitamin D, to make bile acids to digest fats, to allow for healthy neurological function, and to repair and protect cells. It is likely to rise as a part of <u>any</u> healing process within the body.

"For many people, cholesterol drugs may not do any good. For the majority of patients who don't have heart disease, there is no benefit. For people over the age of 65, no matter how much their cholesterol declines, there are no benefits; and there is no benefit in women of any age. The way our healthcare system runs, it is not based on data, it is based on what makes money." ~ Business Week, cover story, January 17, 2008

There is a small reduction in the number of heart attacks for middle-age men taking statins in clinical trials. However, the fact that statins lower cholesterol, but can't be proven to reduce the risk of heart disease, is the thorn in the side of the drug manufacturers. It has yet to be proven that the reduction of heart attacks and mortality are directly influenced by the reduction of cholesterol. In fact, the opposite is true. "Most people are taking something with no chance of benefit" but a proven risk of harm which includes liver failure, muscle wasting, headaches, digestive disorders and nausea. Cholesterol-lowering medications not only provide false hope but are clinically hazardous to your health.

Fortunately, the Maximized Living Nutrition Plans provides much that you can do naturally to prevent the true problem associated with cholesterol, namely the <u>oxidation</u> of cholesterol that is caused by sugar and damaged fats and prevented by healthy fats.

FrankenFood

When you ingest real food, in its natural state, your digestive system will easily break it down, distribute the nutrients to body cells, and quickly eliminate leftover toxins and by-products. No "dis-ease" is created or developed.

Meanwhile, the Food and Drug Administration (FDA) currently approves of approximately 3,000 food additives, preservatives, and colorings that may help food taste better, last longer, and look more appealing. However, when these substances are added, the original nutritional value of these foods is forever altered. Some experts estimate that the average person ingests 140-150 pounds of additives every year, which do not occur in nature or enhance any function in your body. On the contrary, when these chemicals enter your internal ecosystem, they create an imbalance in your body that elicits dangerous side effects. The further away a food is from its natural form, the less efficiently the digestive system can break it down, if at all. Ineffective digestion poisons the body and interferes with its function and healing. In other words, ineffective digestion causes poor health, sickness, and disease.

While hard to believe, many of today's fad diets actually endorse the consumption of foods loaded with additives, preservatives, and colorings. These fad programs use un-natural and prepackaged foods containing processed animal products, chemical-laden powders, meal replacements, and specific stimulant supplements. Although these products may result in short-term weight loss, and in rare cases, long-term, there is no question that they absolutely will <u>not</u> produce a healthy body. On the other hand, eating for good health rather than for weight-loss would not only ensure long-term weight loss success but would help you reach your goals with much less effort.

Making its food ingredients available to customers, a popular fast-food chain has listed its strawberry milkshake ingredients on its Web site. While some might think that strawberries and milk would provide nutritional value, think again:

Strawberry Milkshake: Amyl acetate, amyl butyrate, amyl valerate, anethol, anisyl formate, benzyl acetate, benzyl isobutyrate, butyric acid, cinnamyl isobutyrate, cinnamyl valerate, cognac essential oil, diacetyl, dipropyl ketone, ethyl acetate, ethyl amylketone, ethyl butyrate, ethyl cinnamate, ethyl heptanoate, ethyl heptylate, ethyl lactate, ethyl methylphenylglycidate, ethyl nitrate, ethyl propionate ethyl valerate, heliotropin, hydroxyphrenyl-2-butanone (10% solution in alcohol), ionone, isobuyly anthranilate, isobutyl butyrate, lemon essential oil, maltol, 4-methylacetophenone, methyl anthranilate, methyl benzoate, methyl cinnamate, methyl heptine carbonate, methyl naphthyl ketone, methyl salicylate, mint essential oil, neroli essential oil, nerolin, neryl isobutyrate, orris butter, phenothyl alcohol, rose, rum ether, undecalactone, vanillin, and solvent.

That's right: **There are no strawberries, no milk,** but many chemicals. If you don't know what an ingredient is, you had better find out — your life and health depend on it.

"Safe" Standards

While this fast-food chain publicly lists these ingredients, many additives enter the food system without notice. The FDA does not require food manufacturers to list the ingredients of their additives as long as they are categorized as "Generally Regarded as Safe" or "GRAS." This industry standard merely requires a panel of "experts" to provide a stamp of approval based on scientific evaluation and/or user-based experiences. If an isolated additive has been used in any food without apparent adverse reactions, it can be approved. Certainly, some of these additives may pass the test for harmlessness when used short-term or in moderation. Unfortunately, there is no required test to evaluate for long-term use or for the dangers associate with the cumulative effect of these 3,000 chemicals. It would be safe to say that your body would be better off without them than with them, even in small amounts.

While the body has multiple protective mechanisms for ridding itself of toxins and restoring harmony, it has its limitations. Dr. Paula Baillie-Hamilton, author of *The Detox Diet*, proposes that our own natural weight-control system is being poisoned by toxic chemicals that we encounter every day in foods and household products. Because toxins are fat-soluble, the body naturally creates fat to safely store those toxins and protect the body — this fat cannot be burned off on the treadmill. Toxic fat will block the processing of other nutrients, rob your energy, contaminate your cells, affect moods, and contribute to every type of symptom and disease known to humanity.

Pesticides: On Your Lawn and in Your Food

Approximately 3 million tons of pesticides are used each year worldwide. More than 1,600 chemicals are used to produce pesticides, most of which have not been tested for their toxic effects on humans. Pesticides are toxic by design — they are used to kill insects, fungi, rodents, weeds, and other nuisances to food production. They are known to be toxic inside the human body as well.

A report released by the Pesticide Action Network of North America (PANNA) found that Americans can receive up to 70 daily exposures to residues of "persistent organic pollutants" through their diets alone. Persistent organic pollutants include dioxin, DDT, PCBs, and other known hazards to human health. Children are the most vulnerable due to their size and the fact that they are in the developmental phases of their lives.

Exposure to pesticides has been linked to the following:

• Nervous system disorders
• Immune system suppression
• Cancer
• Diabetes
• Reproductive damage
• Hormonal problems and asthma
• Exacerbation of ADD/ADHD/Autism symptoms
• Migraines/Headaches
• Growth and developmental delays

Carbamates are a group of insecticides and herbicides used in the growing of food to kill bugs. Ironically, they also are used as growth promoters in battery-farm situations because they slow down an animal's metabolic rate. Yes, that's right: **The same chemicals used on fruits and vegetables to kill pests are also used to fatten livestock.** Naturally, these chemicals fatten up humans as well.

Note: You will not find a list of pesticides on your food labels. So, you must take every measure possible to avoid potential exposures. If cost is a concern, prioritize your purchases by buying conventional produce that typically has a lower pesticide load. Items with higher toxic loads should be the first on your list to buy organic. Refer to the Environmental Working Group's "Clean Fifteen" and "Dirty Dozen" on page 79.

Monosodium Glutamate (MSG)

Once associated exclusively with Chinese food, MSG is in more foods than you would imagine. Typical offenders include flavored snack chips, flavored deli meats, soups, coffee, and prepackaged rice and pasta mixes. This chemical additive enhances flavor and keeps you coming back for more. Unfortunately, it is classified as an excitotoxin and is known to stimulate nerve cells to the point of death. Excitotoxins are capable of crossing the blood-brain barrier and cause further damage within the brain.

The symptoms associated with MSG include headaches, migraines, sterility, cancer, mood swings, depression, hyperactivity, asthma, heart irregularities, and endocrine disruptions. MSG drives cholesterol into the blood vessel walls. By stimulating the production of free radicals, a single dose of MSG has been shown to result in higher concentrations of free radicals in the body — for life!

Warning: MSG is often disguised on food labels as hydrolyzed vegetable protein, yeast extract, autolyzed yeast, or sodium caseinate. Check the labels carefully.

Nitrites (Sodium Nitrite)

Nitrites are associated mostly with packaged meat, because they give a red, "fresh" color to hot dogs, deli meats, bacon, sausage, pepperoni, salami, beef jerky, and even frozen foods and canned soups that contain red meat. When ingested, nitrites form cancer-causing nitrosamines.

Nitrites are banned in many countries. At one time, they were about to be banned from use in the United States, until pressure from the meat industry halted the initiative. In 2009, the World Cancer Research Fund (WCRF) published its review of more than 7,000 clinical studies of the relationships between diet and cancer. The WCRF's most startling statement: **Processed meats are too dangerous for human consumption.**

Another large-scale study of nitrites in processed meats tracked 200,000 people over a seven-year period and published its results in 2005. The University of Hawaii's lead researcher, Ute Nothlings, found the consumption of processed meats containing nitrites increased the risk of pancreatic cancer by 67 percent.

Unfortunately, the corporations that dominate American food and agricultural interests hold tremendous influence over the FDA and U.S. Department of Agriculture (USDA); and as a result, nitrites remain in packaged meats. Consumers are offered no great protection — other than becoming educated and making informed decisions.

Chemical Bleaching of Flour

If the glycemic action of white flour wasn't enough of a health concern, the process in which this flour becomes "white" poses an additional hazard to your health. To whiten the flour, mills use various chemical bleaches, including the oxide of nitrogen, chlorine, chloride, nitrosyl and benzoyl peroxide, mixed with various chemical salts.

Bleached flour is yet another reason to stick with whole grains.

Growth Hormone and Antibiotics

Eric Schlosser exposes in his book *Fast Food Nation* that "the old meatpacking plants in Chicago slaughtered about 50 cattle an hour. Twenty years ago, new plants in the High Plains slaughtered about 175 cattle an hour. Today some plants slaughter up to 400 cattle an hour — about half a dozen animals every minute."

In order to slaughter such a high number of cattle every minute, animals are packed into feedlots, fed pesticide-sprayed grain to fatten them up quickly, and administered steroid hormones to accelerate growth. Not following their natural diet or exercise patterns, cattle often fall ill and require antibiotics just to be kept alive. The same is true for chickens that are mass-produced for worldwide delivery.

Hormone residues in commercially-raised meat can go on to disrupt hormones in humans who consume them. Hormone residues in beef have been implicated in the early onset of puberty in girls, which put them at greater risk of developing breast cancer and other forms of cancer. Children, pregnant women, and the unborn are thought to be most susceptible to the negative health effects of hormone residues, which may include developmental problems, reproductive system disorders, and an increased risk of developing breast, prostate, and colon cancer.

Residues of the antibiotics used to treat livestock are known carcinogens and allergens when passed on to humans. Perhaps the greatest danger associated with the consumption of these antibiotics is that they cause a buildup of antibiotic-resistant super-germs in the animals. When these resistant bacteria are consumed by people, they are exposed to pathogens that stress the immune system beyond its normal capacity.

Quit Counting Calories — Start Counting Chemicals

Even the smallest amount of synthetic chemicals directly damage muscles and distort hormones that control muscular growth. Dr. Richie Shoemaker has written that weight loss has little to do with caloric intake or exercise but "is actually about hormones such as insulin, leptin, and others they control."

The body's leptin levels not only go out of balance due to Standard North American Diet patterns but also in response to toxins that ultimately destroy the leptin receptors in your brain. Not even daily exercise and the cleanest diet will reshape a person's physique when toxins enter into the mix.

Ultimately, the concern about toxins entering into the body goes beyond obesity. There are millions of thin people every year who get cancer, heart disease, diabetes, and autoimmune disorders without any "conventional" explanation.

Food regulators continue to permit "acceptable" doses of toxic chemicals in today's foods. How long these chemicals will be allowed in our food supply is a guessing game. While they may be "generally regarded as safe" for the time being, it is not uncommon for the leading scientific study of today to be refuted tomorrow. Trusting your diet to the science of the day can be a dangerous gamble for you and your family's health. Sticking to the original design, as described in the following pages, is a fail-proof plan that not only does not involve risks, but will allow you to live life abundantly and in good health.

Chapter 2

Where are You?

Take this short quiz to see where you currently stand in terms of your diet and eating habits.

☑ Do you eat out more than three times per week?

☐ Do you eat boxed foods more than twice per week?

☐ Do you drink any type of soda?

☑ Do you eat less than five servings of vegetables per day?

☑ Do you drink less than four glasses of water per day?

☑ Do you feel "addicted" to certain foods?

☑ Do you typically opt for lower-fat and lower-calorie foods when given the choice?

☑ Do you eat white flour, white rice, or white bread?

☐ Do you use artificial sweeteners, such as aspartame, Splenda®, and NutraSweet®, or consume foods that contain them?

☐ Do you eat fried foods more than once per week?

☑ Do you eat processed "deli" meat, bacon, sausage, or hot dogs?

☑ Do you think that you get all your needed nutrients from food and therefore pass on supplements, including multivitamins and fish oil?

☑ Do you use canola oil or vegetable oils in cooking or in salad dressings?

☑ Do you use margarine?

☑ Are most of the fruits and vegetables you eat conventionally grown (non-organic)?

☑ Do you consume milk and dairy products that are purchased from the grocery store?

☑ Are the majority of your animal products purchased from the meat counter or freezer at the grocery store (as opposed to a health food store or local farmer)?

☑ Do you consider price and convenience of food to be more important than nutritional quality?

☐ Do you eat sweets or candy more than once per week?

☐ Do you drink more than 3 alcoholic beverages per week?

☑ Do you eat while rushed or under stress?

☐ Do you, your doctor, or family think that you need to lose some body fat?

☐ Do you have irregular blood sugar, diabetes, or pre-diabetes?

☐ Do you have blood pressure over 120/80?

☑ Do you suffer from sinus conditions, asthma, or allergies (including rashes, eczema, or hives)?

☑ Do you have gastrointestinal concerns?

☑ Do you frequently experience fatigue or insomnia?

☐ Do you have emotional/mental challenges or trouble concentrating?

☑ Do you suffer from joint pain or muscle aches?

☐ Do you have hormonal imbalances?

Tally the number of items you checked above and mark your score below.

Total = 14

Where Do You Stand and Where Do You Start?

0-5 GREAT

You are obviously a nutritionally conscious person and are off to a good start! Like most of us, you may need to make some minor improvements to your nutrition plans. We trust the core principles of the Maximized Living Nutrition Plans described in this book will help you take your health to the next level.

6-10 GOOD

You are doing pretty well but likely need stronger discipline with your eating habits. If you can target and stick to the basic principles of the Core Plan, you will likely experience speedy improvements in your health.

11-15 IMPROVEMENT NEEDED

Your diet needs some work — although you may not realize it. It's quite likely that you are doing your best, following other food guides, and counting calories. But according to the principles of Maximized Living, you are probably doing some harm to your health. You will probably learn some surprising things in the Maximized Living Nutrition Plans that contradict traditional wisdom. Rather than becoming overwhelmed, take small steps. You can deal with these one at a time. Be sure to identify any conditions listed in Chapter 4 that make you a candidate for the Advanced Plan, which you may need to follow in order to reach your health goals. Small successes can get you motivated to make more changes. Aim to get your score below 6 within six months.

16-20 PRE-DISEASE

Whether you realize it or not, your eating habits will not be without serious health consequences. If you haven't already started to experience symptoms, or have not yet been diagnosed with any disease, that day is around the corner if immediate changes are not made. Fortunately, your score is low enough that following the Advanced Plan will help you reduce your score even further — and improve your health significantly — within six months' time. However, long-standing illness or other factors described in Chapter 4 may prolong your recovery. You will probably feel poorly in your first few weeks of changes; but once your body adapts, you will undoubtedly feel the positive effects, like so many Maximized Living participants across the globe.

21+ CRISIS

It is time to pull out all of the stops. Whether or not your doctor has diagnosed it, you are in a serious state of health crisis and are moving in the wrong direction. The Advanced Plan is designed to help you reverse the track you are on. Start making changes and moving in the right direction today. The longer you wait, the less likely you will ever start. Even if you begin slowly, just get started. You are better off moving in the right direction slowly than the wrong direction quickly.

As you may have guessed, all of the items on the list are problematic when it comes to being healthy. After all, the ideal score is "zero." It is imperative that you be able to avoid answering yes to most of them. A score of 30 out of 30 would go to someone following the Standard North American Diet religiously. It is sad but true that North Americans hold the dubious honor of having the worst diets on the planet and the most lifestyle-related diseases, such as heart disease, diabetes, high blood pressure, and cancer.

Every person will at some point in their lifetime decide to make — and have to make — their own health their top priority. We trust you will make this decision today — not tomorrow.

Regardless of your starting point, everyone has room to improve. Nutrition, just like life, is a marathon, not a sprint. Let's get started.

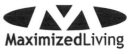

MaximizedLiving

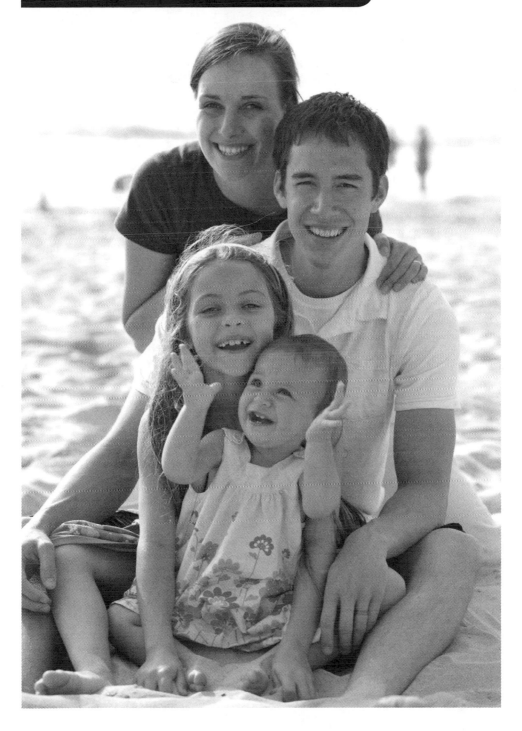

Chapter 3

The Core Plan ◉

The Three Core Principles

Most North Americans need to make several changes in order to prevent and reverse disease and illness. The Three Core Principles are the foundation for the Nutrition Plans, regardless of one's age, genetic background, or medical history. They are broken down by food group: fats, protein, and carbohydrates.

THE CORE PLAN

Fat

Healthy fats vs. damaged fats:

Eat more healthy fats; eliminate all damaged fats.

Protein

Naturally raised vs. unnaturally raised animals:

Go organic and natural for animals because these are at the top of the food chain.

Carbohydrates

Whole carbohydrates vs. refined carbohydrates:

Eat more vegetables — eliminate refined grains and sugars.

FOOD CHOICES

Fat

The number one missing ingredient in the standard North American diet is not a vitamin or mineral but good fat. Be sure to eat good fats with every meal. They are essential to hormone production, cancer prevention, metabolism regulation, fat-burning, brain development, weight loss, cellular healing, and anti-inflammation.

Bad fats, such as hydrogenated and partially-hydrogenated oils, trans fats, and rancid vegetable oils, are linked to cellular congestion and are related to cancer, heart disease, and neurotoxicity. Bad fats also are linked to chronic inflammation, which is the underlying cause of 21st-century diseases and the leading disease killers in North America.

HEALTHY FATS FOR THE CORE PLAN

Raw Nuts and Seeds	
Almonds	Cashews
Flaxseed	Hemp Seed
Pecans	Pine Nuts
Macadamia Nuts	Sesame Seeds
Sunflower Seeds	Walnuts
Raw Nut and Seed Butters (almond butter, macadamia butter, and raw tahini)	

Animal Proteins with Good Fats	
Grass-Fed Meat	contains good fats in the ideal ratio for consumption
Fish	best are cold-water fish (salmon, mahi-mahi, mackerel, halibut) and/ or smaller fish on the food chain (sardines, anchovies)
Eggs	from hens who are cage-free/free-range, organic, hormone-free/antibiotic-free, and fed no animal by-products

Full Fat Dairy Products
Full-fat, organic dairy is a bare minimum. Non-homogenized is even better. Non-pasteurized (raw) is best, if available. Dairy products with reduced fat contain a higher percentage of sugar.

Full-Fat Raw Milk	Cream
Full-Fat Plain Yogurt	Raw Cheeses
Butter (preferably raw)	Kefir
Ghee (clarified butter)	

Oils

Acceptable for Heat	Do Not Heat
Coconut Oil (best for high heat)	Walnut, Flaxseed, Avocado Oil
Grape Seed Oil	Cod Liver Oil
Olive Oil (medium heat only – do not let it smoke)	Hemp Seed Oil (good fats in the right ratio)

Other

Olives	Avocado	Coconut products: milk, oil, butter, flakes, flesh, flour and spreads

Grain-Free Carbohydrate Replacements

Flax seed bread, muffins, and crackers	These good-fat snacks replace traditional, homemade, unhealthy carbohydrates. Explore the recipes starting on page 104.
Almond flour cookies	

Special Focus: Dairy

It is estimated that 44 percent of the beverages consumed by those under 18 are dairy products. However, the consumption of dairy products is one of the most controversial topics in the world of health and wellness.

- The government food guides advise that you consume two to four servings of milk products per day.

- Hundreds of wellness authors throughout the years have advised against dairy consumption.

- Authors who support the Paleolithic diet suggest that there is little or no harm with respect to the consumption of dairy.

- Some vegetarian plans not allowing meat will permit eggs and dairy.

- Many nutritionists agree that dairy is one of the more common allergens seen today and suggest that most people are allergic to milk, citing the lack of human enzymes to digest lactose (dairy sugar) after puberty. As you will see, dairy products are listed in a number of recipes and food choices within the Nutrition Plans . While these recipes and food choices may refer exclusively to "dairy," we advise you to note that not all dairy products – and not all people – are created equal.

Genetic Differences

It is thought that people of northern European genetic descent are typically more susceptible to the ill effects that dairy products cause in the digestive system. It also has been observed that cultures in the Middle East and in Africa, who have survived on dairy as a major part of their diets for centuries, do not seem to suffer the rampant negative effects that nutrition authors suggest should be the norm.

While all humans' production of the enzymes necessary to break down lactose decreases after puberty, some individuals' gastrointestinal systems have a better tolerance for the large proteins that are contained in cow's milk.

Those who genetically tolerate dairy at the gastrointestinal level will do better with dairy products than others. Keep in mind that the process of identifying your genetic type may not be self-evident. Therefore, digestive hypersensitivity testing by a certified laboratory is the most reliable test for those who are uncertain.

Milk's Natural State

When the Masai were studied and observed to be free of heart disease, yet surviving on the full-fat milk of their cows, they were consuming dairy in its natural state – raw.

The overwhelming majority of today's commercial dairy is not raw but pasteurized and homogenized. Pasteurization heats milk to a temperature below the boiling point to reduce the number of pathogenic micro-organisms that may be present in the original raw milk. While the purpose of pasteurization is to destroy pathogens, pasteurization also destroys the vitamins, fats, and proteins touted as the beneficial nutrients you need. It is for this reason you will often see nutrients, including calcium and vitamin D, added back into dairy products or "fortified" post-pasteurization. Unfortunately, healthy fats and proteins which have been "de-natured" through the heating process cannot be "re-natured;" and as a result, they are left in dairy products in damaged forms. Heat also inactivates the beneficial bacteria found in raw milk, which would otherwise prevent pathogens like salmonella from proliferating. In fact, most salmonella outbreaks linked to milk stem from fully pasteurized and homogenized milk, not raw milk.

Homogenization of milk breaks the fat particles into smaller sizes to prevent the natural separation of cream to the top of the solution. This allows for the sale of non-separating 1 percent, 2 percent, and whole milk. These altered and compressed fat particles can be absorbed easily into the blood stream along with toxic dairy enzymes, while in their natural form they would have passed through the digestive system unabsorbed. It is the assimilation of these de-natured and toxic components — that would otherwise be excreted out of the human — which displace the essential human proteins that keep arteries healthy.

Dairy cattle, forced to produce more milk than is natural, are exposed to high levels of growth hormones and are susceptible to illness. They are administered antibiotics for most of their lives. The residues of antibiotics end up in the food chain, along with growth hormones, which have been linked to premature development, particularly in girls.

Skim Milk

Skim milk is another win for the low-fat craze. Skim milk has a higher ratio of milk sugar with respect to milk fat and presents the same problems as other foods high in sugar. Furthermore, skim milk is even more processed than whole milk. Every extra step of processing is another step away from the natural state. A one-year study of more than 12,000 children ages 9-14 found that the more milk children drank, the more weight they gained. The majority of children in the study were drinking skim milk.

Osteoporosis

Osteoporosis is not due to a lack of calcium. Osteoporosis is caused by a negative calcium balance in the blood that is due to high acidity and higher levels of unhealthy minerals, including phosphates that cause calcium depletion from its storage site: bones. Since osteoporosis is highest in parts of the world where dairy is a daily staple, it should be clear that the consumption of more dairy to "prevent" osteoporosis is wishful thinking. To get all the calcium you need in its healthy state your body can use, go for spinach, broccoli, cauliflower, salmon, sardines, figs, baked beans, brazil nuts, walnuts, almonds, kelp, and honeydew melons.

Where to Start

If you can be certain that your genetic type is compatible with dairy, look for dairy in its purest form: raw, full-fat, and non-homogenized. Since dairy is an animal product, always buy organic, consistent with the principles of toxic bioaccumulation described on page 38.

Because raw dairy is banned in many states, you may not have this option. At a bare minimum, look for organic, non-homogenized, full-fat dairy products. Full-fat and organic dairy products are the minimal requirements on the Maximized Living Nutrition Planss. Consuming organic dairy, at a bare minimum, will assure that your dairy is free from dangerous hormones and antibiotics. Moderate your intake and monitor your tolerance.

If you cannot be certain that your genetic type is compatible with dairy, don't panic. The majority of your fluids should come from water. And like cows, you'll get plenty of calcium and nutrients from fresh vegetation.

Alternatives

If you are allergic or intolerant to dairy — or choose to limit your consumption — know that you have many options. Coconut milk and unsweetened almond milk can be used in most recipes calling for milk. Many recipes calling for cheese can do without. Numerous regions allow raw cheese to be sold in stores, even where raw milk is banned.

Notes: Those with allergies or intolerances typically find that hard cheeses cause fewer digestive problems than soft cheeses do and that healthy whey protein also is safe to consume. Raw, grass-fed whey protein excludes the casein component of dairy that is most often the culprit of sensitivities in the gut.

Special Focus: Coconut

North Americans have been taught to fear coconut because it is high in fat, high in calories, and because coconut oil contains 91 percent saturated fat. Accordingly, with the traditional lipid hypothesis, heart patients have been advised to shy away from any foods that might raise cholesterol due to saturated fat content. These foods include coconut, cashew, animal fat, and butter.

Yet, studies of Polynesian and Sri Lankan populations, where coconut consumption is high, have found that "dietary coconut oil does not lead to high serum cholesterol nor to high coronary heart disease mortality, or morbidity." Further studies on atherosclerosis and coconut consumption have found "no change in serum cholesterol level from coconut oil." It turns out that the earlier studies linking coconut products to heart disease were studying hydrogenated coconut oil. The vegetable oil industry, tied closely with the FDA, has propagated this erroneous research for decades.

As discussed in Chapter 1, the labeling of all saturated fats as "unhealthy" is a misnomer. There are healthy saturated fats and there are damaged saturated fats. When animals are fed grain, their antioxidants are depleted and their fats become more susceptible to oxidation and damage. When coconut fat or even animal fat is consumed in its purest form, the saturated fat is protected from oxidation by abundant antioxidants and offers incredible health benefits.

Because saturated fats are medium-chain, (not longer-chain), fatty acids, most of the saturated fat in coconut oil is readily usable by the human body. The larger the fatty acids the more energy is required by the body to break them down. For this reason, coconut is converted into quick energy and less likely to be stored as fat or cause obesity. Shown to support the thyroid, heart, and immune system, coconut is one of the healthiest foods in the world today.

Damaged Fats to Eliminate on the Core Plan

- Hydrogenated and partially-hydrogenated oils
- Rancid oils (corn oil, vegetable oil, canola oil, cottonseed oil, soybean oil, safflower oil, and sunflower oil)
- Trans fats (margarine, synthetic butters, and shortening)
- Roasted nuts and seeds
- Roasted nut and seed butters
- Pasteurized and homogenized dairy products

Protein

Countless studies link commercial meats with cancer and heart disease. In contrast, naturally raised meats provide nutrients, fatty acids, and amino acids that are essential for good health. Many cultures, along with our own Paleolithic ancestors, have survived on naturally-raised meats without experiencing cancer or heart disease in the proportions we do in North America.

To avoid and/or reduce the toxic burden of harmful nutrients in your body, purchase organic and natural, especially for animals at the top of the food chain. (See below for further explanation)

> **TIP: You aren't what you eat. You are what you are eating ate.**

Toxic Bioaccumulation

When a potentially toxic and non-biodegradable substance, such as a pesticide or herbicide, is released into the environment, its concentration may be so low that it causes no obvious damage. It may move into plants at the same low concentration in which it exists in water or soil. However, an herbivore, (a plant-eating animal), must eat about 10 grams of living matter to make 1 gram of itself. So herbivores will on average take in as much of the potentially toxic substance as is found in 10 individual plants. A carnivore, (a meat-eating animal), will accumulate the toxin to a concentration about 10 times that found in an herbivore, or 100 times that found in individual soils and plants. Animals at the top of the food chain may contain toxic compounds in the most damaging concentration of all, even though the concentration in the environment or in other species may be too low to cause harm.

Fatty Acid Ratio Distortion

When red-meat animals that would naturally eat grass are fed grain, their fatty acid ratios are altered and their good saturated fats are denatured, becoming bad fats. As a result, they become susceptible to sickness and disease and require a constant dose of antibiotics.

Grass-fed and free-range meats provide many of the fatty acids that are missing in the Standard North American Diet (arachidonic acid, conjugated linoleic acid and the proper ratio of omega-6 to omega-3 fatty acids), which your body actually needs to burn fat, to detoxify, and to prevent heart disease and cancer.

Good Proteins for the Core Plan

Animal Proteins	
Grass-fed Meat (beef, lamb)	Contains good fats in the ideal ratio for consumption. Choose grass-fed, free-range, cage-free, and hormone-free animal sources.
Fish	Best are cold-water fish (salmon, mahi-mahi, mackerel, halibut), from the cleanest waters (Pacific and Alaskan oceans), and those that are lowest on the food chain (sardines, anchovies)
Eggs	From hens that are cage-free/free-range, organic, hormone-free/antibiotic-free, and fed no animal byproducts
Poultry	Naturally-raised, free-range, hormone-free/antibiotic-free poultry (chicken, turkey)

Raw Nuts and Seeds

These are an excellent source of protein and substitute for meat products.
Almonds, cashews, flaxseed, hemp seeds, pecans, pine nuts, macadamia nuts, sesame seeds, sunflower seeds, walnuts, and others. For best results, soak the nuts and seeds overnight in filtered water. Then drain, dry, and store in glass jars in the refrigerator. This releases the natural enzymes and makes them easier to digest and assimilate.

Fermented Soy Products		
Miso	Tempeh	Tamari

Dairy Products

These are an excellent source of protein and substitute for meat products.
Full-fat, organic dairy is a bare minimum. Non-homogenized is even better.
Non-pasteurized (raw) is best, if available.
Dairy products with reduced fat contain a higher percentage of sugar.
Full-fat raw milk, full-fat plain yogurt, raw cheeses, kefir, whey protein

> **Protein tip:** Have some protein with every meal, and most importantly when your body needs it most (toward the end of the day and thirty to forty-five minutes after exercise).

Bad Proteins to Eliminate

- Grain-fed red meats (beef, lamb)
- Pork (highly acidic and large toxic load)
- Conventionally raised poultry (chicken, turkey)
- Farm-raised fish (these fish are fed grains, which is not their natural diet, and they are not raised humanely)
- Shellfish (highly acidic; large toxic load) and large ocean fish (tuna, cod)
- Processed soy products (tofu, soy nuts, soy milk, and soy formula)
- Whey protein (hydrolyzed, treated with heat and/or from pasteurized dairy)
- Roasted nuts and seeds (highly acidic, loss of nutrients; heat turns natural oils rancid)
- Pasteurized and homogenized dairy products

Special Focus: Pork and Shellfish

Notable on the list of bad proteins to eliminate are pork and shellfish. This can be difficult to swallow (in more ways than one!) because pork and shellfish make up some of North America's favorite Western dishes:

Bacon	Pepperoni	Clams	Mussels
Ham	Ribs	Oysters	Scallops
Pork chops	Crab	Lobster	

Consistent with the principle of toxic bioaccumulation, it is vital that when switching to healthier foods you start with animal proteins. Pork and shellfish are the ultimate scavengers — they consume waste and excrement. Shellfish, by design, clean the waste of the polluted ocean floor. Pigs will eat sick, infected animals — even their own dead young.

All syndromes of shellfish poisoning, whether acute or latent, share common features. Shellfish toxins are water-soluble, and heat- and acid-stable. So the toxins are not inactivated by ordinary cooking methods. Therefore, even if you don't experience acute symptoms of "food poisoning," you are undoubtedly stockpiling the toxins without knowing it.

Neither group of animals has a digestive system that is sophisticated enough to effectively process and eliminate toxins. The pig's gastrointestinal tract moves food through its system in just four hours, and doesn't have any sophisticated method of filtering and eliminating toxins. Furthermore, pigs may have sweat glands; but they do not sweat efficiently. That's why Wilbur sits in the mud to cool down. Without effective sweating, the toxins that accumulate in the meat, fat, and skin of the pig are much less likely to be eliminated.

When compared with other animals acceptable on the Maximized Living Nutrition Plans, such as beef, lamb and poultry, you will note that these animals have systems of digestion and elimination (including sweating through the skin) that are close to those found in humans. Similarly, they take up to 24 hours to process, filter, and eliminate toxins. These animals inherently assimilate only the important nutrients from their meals. Unlike pork and shellfish, animals such as beef, lamb, poultry, and wild game thrive on fresh vegetation — not waste products — as their source of food.

Special Focus: Soy

Soy has been touted as a super health food for the past several decades, partly by the "vegetarian movement," which has blessed us with soy hot dogs, soy hamburgers, soy milk, and even soy ice cream. And don't forget about soy cheese, soy cereal, soy nuts, soy nuggets and tofu (processed soy). But have you ever considered where soy comes from in the first place? The soy bean is indeed a natural food, but it has become one of the most genetically modified crops in the industry. Furthermore, in countries where soy beans grow naturally and wild, soy is never the main course as it is here for so many consumers trying to eat "healthy."

The reality is that soy has a dark side — and the majority of health-conscious consumers eating modernized soy products are eating "food" that was never designed for human consumption. Fermented soy is the exception. Those foods would include tamari, miso, tempeh, amakaze, and natto that are acceptable on the Maximized Living Nutrition Plans but still should not be considered one's primary food source. The reality is that you won't find miso cheese or miso milk in any grocery store. The fermentation actually helps negate some of soy's harmful effects described below.

Remember: The soy business has become a major industry worth big bucks to manufacturers, so soy products continue to expand. Soybean oil, which is used in thousands of salad dressings, may go rancid in the body; but it is cheap and low in saturated fat. You will continue to see it on the label of many products, but please look beyond the "healthy" label.

Dr. Kaayla Daniel, author of *the Whole Soy Story,* explains:

- Soybeans are high in natural toxins, also known as "anti-nutrients". This includes a large quantity of inhibitors that deter the enzymes needed for protein digestion. These enzyme inhibitors are not entirely disabled during ordinary cooking. The result is extensive gastric distress and chronic deficiencies in amino acid uptake, which can result in pancreatic impairment and cancer.

- Soybeans contain hemaglutinin, which causes red blood cells to clump together. Soybeans also have growth-depressant substances. And while these substances are reduced in processing, they are not completely eliminated.

- Soy contains goitrogens, which frequently lead to depressed thyroid function.

- Most soybeans are high in phytates, which prevent the absorption of minerals, including calcium, magnesium, iron, and zinc, all of which are co-factors for optimal biochemistry in the body. Eating meat reduces the mineral-blocking effects of these phytates, and so it is helpful if you do eat soy to also eat meat.

- Finally, in an effort to remove the anti-nutrients from soy, soybeans are taken through a series of chemical processes, including acid washing in aluminum tanks. This leaches high levels of aluminum, a toxic heavy metal, into the final soy products. Many soy foods also have toxic levels of manganese. Soy formula has up to eighty times higher manganese than is found in human breast milk.

The mass genetic modification of soy brings with it a host of additional concerns, which include, but are not limited to the following: intestinal damage, allergies, sterility, liver damage, pancreatic damage, kidney damage, increased inflammation, DNA disruption (that's a scary one), increased toxicity, and endocrine disruptions. Because the phytonutrients in soy mimic estrogen in the body, and because studies have shown that the risks are greatest in children, some countries are starting to ban or limit the availability of soy "foods" for babies and children — particularly for boys.

There are much better protein sources and alternatives to dairy than turning to soy. As always in Maximized Living, look to foods in the state they were designed for human consumption, not modified in processed and packaged foods.

Carbohydrates

Carbohydates, like fruits, vegetables, and grains, are energy-producing foods. The higher a carbohydrate is on the glycemic index, the quicker it turns into sugar and upsets your hormone cycles.

The reality is that sugar is everywhere. According to published reports, the number one source of sugar for the vast majority of North Americans is soft drinks. (*San Mateo County Times.*)   Other sources include: lunch meats, pizza, sauces, breads, soups, crackers, fruit drinks, canned foods, yogurt, ketchup, and mayonnaise. Read the ingredients; you will be shocked. Today, North Americans consume an average of 120 pounds of sugar per year per person compared to five pounds per year per family in the early 1900s. (Robbins, *Healthy at 100.*)

As stated above, remember that refined carbohydrates, such as flour, bread, and rice, turn into sugar almost immediately after putting them in your mouth and your saliva starts breaking them down. Don't be fooled. These foods are still sugar even if they don't taste sweet.

Sugar is also an "anti-nutrient." Not only does it include an insignificant amount of vitamins and minerals, it actually robs your body of precious nutrient stores. The herb stevia is the preferred alternative sweetener. Xylitol is an acceptable alternate. While alternatives like honey and maple syrup are "natural," they will spike blood sugar considerably.

High glycemic and refined sugars cause elevated glucose, which in turn elevates insulin, leading to premature aging and degenerative disease (type 2 diabetes, heart disease, inflammation of the arteries, and cancer).

Therefore, the only grains acceptable on the Maximized Living Core Nutrition Plans are those that are sprouted, whole-grain, or stone-ground.

Lower-Glycemic Carbohydrates
High in fiber, these are always your best carbohydrate choices any time of the day.

Moderate-Glycemic Carbohydrates
Reduce consumption of these carbohydrates after lunch.
Completely eliminate these carbohydrates after lunch if weight loss is a concern.

High-Glycemic Carbohydrates
Eat these carbohydrates only during recovery from exercise.
Avoid them completely if weight loss is a concern.

Refined Carbohydrates
Sugars and refined grains are eliminated completely on the
Maximized Living Nutrition Plans.

Good Carbohydrates for the Core Plan

High-Fiber/Low-Glycemic Carbohydrates
High in fiber, these are always your best carbohydrate choices any time of the day.

Vegetables		
Arugula	Asparagus	Bamboo Shoots
Bean Sprouts	Beet Greens	Bell Peppers (red, yellow, green)
Broadbeans	Broccoli	Brussel Sprouts
Cabbage	Cassava	Cauliflower

Vegetables		
Celery	Chayote Fruit	Chicory
Chives	Collard Greens	Coriander
Cucumber	Dandelion Greens	Eggplant
Endive	Fennel	Garlic
Ginger Root	Green Beans	Heart of Palm
Jicama (raw)	Jalapeno Peppers	Kale
Kohlrabi	Lettuce	Mushrooms
Mustard Greens	Onions	Parsley
Radishes	Radicchio	Snap Beans
Snow Peas	Shallots	Spinach
Spaghetti Squash	Summer Squash	Swiss Chard
Tomatoes	Turnip Greens	Watercress
Zucchini		

Fruits		
Blackberries	Blueberries	Boysenberries
Elderberries	Gooseberries	Loganberries
Raspberries	Strawberries	Lemons
Limes	Granny Smith Apples	

Moderate-Fiber/Moderate-Glycemic Carbohydrates
Reduce consumption of these carbohydrates after lunch.
Completely eliminate these carbohydrates after lunch if weight loss is a concern.

Vegetables and Grains		
Leeks	Lima Beans	Okra
Pumpkin	Sweet Potato or Yam	Turnip
Legumes	Artichokes	Squash (acorn, butternut, winter)
Adzuki Beans	Black Beans	Chick Peas (garbanzo)
Cowpeas	French Beans	Great Northern Beans
Kidney Beans	Lentils	Mung Beans
Navy Beans	Pinto Beans	Split Peas

Vegetables and Grains		
White Beans	Yellow Beans	Barley
Brown Rice	Buckwheat (kasha)	Bulgar (tabouli)
Millet	Rye	Steel Cut Oats
Semolina	Tapioca	Whole Grain Breads
Ezekiel 4:9® Bread	Whole Grains	100% Whole Grain Cooked Cereals and Crackers

Whether or not you are trying to lose weight, healthy grains are best used as an energy source when consumed early in the day. They should not be eaten after lunch.

Fruits		
Cherries	Pear	Fresh Apricots
Melons	Orange	Peaches
Plum	Grapefruit	Pitted Prunes
Apples	Kiwi fruit	Nectarines
Tangerines	Passion Fruit	Persimmons
Pomegranates		

Low-Fiber/High-Glycemic Carbohydrates

Eat these carbohydrates only during recovery from exercise. Avoid them completely if weight loss is a concern.

Fruits		
Banana	Pineapple	Grapes
Watermelon	Mango	Papaya
Dates	Honey	Fruit juice

Vegetables, Tubers and Grains

Be cautious with carbohydrates and sugars from vegetables that are not grown above ground because they will alter insulin levels.

Carrots	Corn	Potatoes
Root Vegetables	Beets	

Special Focus: Raw vs. Cooked Food

The more a food is altered from its natural state, the less benefit it has for your body. While cooking foods is far less invasive than chemically altering them, it should be noted that cooked foods lose vital nutrients and enzymes, which your body needs to survive. Fat, protein, and carbohydrates are essential to support all bodily functions. When heated, these substances become difficult for the body to use effectively.

While it is true that some foods are more susceptible to heat and less likely to become denatured (i.e. coconut oil), we encourage you to strive for more raw foods in your diet. Specifically, we encourage vegetables, because their numerous nutrients and live enzymes, so important for good health, are diminished when heated over 105°F.

Fats should never be heated beyond their smoking point, as this will create substances that become unrecognizable and unusable by your body and will cause elements of the blood to clump together creating disease.

Your body fills up on nutrients – not calories.

Cooked foods offer just as many calories but with fewer nutrients. Raw foods, on the other hand, provide the nutrients that will keep you full longer.

Raw foods are easier on your digestive system

Natural fibers in fruits, vegetables, nuts, and seeds, which sweep the digestive tract clean, change from their natural state in cooked food. As a result, they take longer to move through the digestive tract. The transit time for raw foods is typically 24 to 36 hours whereas cooked foods can take 40 to 100 hours to move through the system. This opens up the door for constipation and fermentation, which create unhealthy waste in the system.

The protein from raw vegetables offers your body the best source of amino acids. Many vegetables have more amino acids per calorie than animal protein. Amino acids, however, are susceptible to damage by heat. Consumption of excess denatured, amino acids will not only cause damage to the lining of the digestive tract, (and thereby produce food sensitivities), but will prevent the body from absorbing the complete amino acids needed to create cells, organs, and tissues, which control all bodily functions.

Experience the energy offered by raw foods

The digestion of food is an exhaustive process on the body. It takes 30 percent of our energy to digest even a raw food meal, but 60 percent of our energy to digest a cooked meal. This is the primary reason why people are energetic after eating a salad or a healthy smoothie but tired after a meal of cooked meat and vegetables — even if the vegetables are organic. Decreased energy interferes with sleep and healing achieved by your body when it is at rest. To wake up with more energy each day, increase the number of raw foods with each meal.

Microwaves vs. the Stovetop?

If you must cook your food, consider using the most natural means. While all methods of heating food are known to lessen its quality, science has shown repeatedly that microwaves, by far, have the worst impact. Whereas lightly steamed broccoli loses 11 percent of its cancer-fighting antioxidants, up to 97 percent can be lost when microwaved. Furthermore, nearly 100 percent of people have food sensitivities to microwaved foods due to their altered chemical composition. An even greater concern is that microwaving causes the leaching of toxins into foods when cooked in plastic dishes. Bisphenol A, a chemical toxin found in plastic known to affect neural and reproductive development, has been banned from baby bottles in Canada — and may soon be banned in the United States — because of its link to cancer, early puberty, obesity, and diabetes. One can avoid the possibility of toxic contamination by choosing natural cooking methods rather than microwaving.

Refined Carbohydrates to Eliminate

Sugar

Sugar promotes yeast growth, lowers the immune system, and alters insulin and hormone levels.

☒ White sugar, brown sugar, molasses

☒ Syrups (maple, rice, corn, and cane varieties)

☒ Dextrose, fructose, glucose, sucrose, maltodextrin. See our Special Focus on Sweeteners below.

☒ Sweetened fruit juice and honey

Refined Grains

If a grain is not "sprouted, whole-grain, or stone-ground," assume it is refined. Caution: Grains that are "untreated, enriched, and unbleached" are not necessarily whole. White bread, white flour, white rice, and white pasta are always refined.

 Special Focus: Sweeteners

When you eliminate refined sugar from your diet, it is natural to go through a seven to fourteen day "withdrawal" period while your taste buds are retrained. You may look to natural sweeteners, which do not elevate blood glucose, insulin, or inflammation.

THE GOOD

Stevia and Xylitol

Stevia is an herb that is 300 times sweeter than sugar in its purest form. It was introduced as a non-caloric table sweetener in the Brazilian market in 1988. Much like any leaf, this herb will not raise blood sugar and is completely natural. Brands come in a variety of tastes and concentrations:

Stevia Conversion Chart

Sugar	Stevia Packets	Stevia Powder	Liquid Stevia
1 teaspoon	½ packet	¼ teaspoon	2 to 3 drops
2 teaspoon	1 packet	½ teaspoon	4 to 6 drops
1 tablespoon	1½ to 2 packet	¾ tablespoons	6 to 9 drops
1 cup	18 to 24 packets	3 to 4 tablespoons	1 teaspoon
2 cups	36 to 48 packets	3 to 4 tablespoons	2 teaspoons

Equivalencies are approximate.

If you can find a "spoonable" or "1-to-1" brand of stevia, equivalencies are not an issue. Just use the 1-to-1 stevia for measure with the amount of sugar in your recipes. These brands are typically bulked up with inulin fiber (from chicory root), erythritol (a fruit crystal), or fructo-oligosaccharides (FOS), which are all acceptable bulking agents. Be cautious of the additive maltodextrin, which is a polysaccharide derived from starch.

If using other brands of stevia, taste test your recipe and adjust the amount of stevia accordingly. Too much stevia may taste bitter. Cinnamon is a helpful addition to reduce bitterness or aftertaste, especially as your tastes change. When substituting stevia for sugar in your own recipes, you may have to adjust for the bulk. Stevia is sold as a nutritional supplement and not as a sweetener or food additive.

Xylitol, a natural sugar alcohol, is also a safe replacement for sugar and will not increase blood sugar. Some people prefer the taste of Xylitol over stevia – this is an individual preference. The main sources of commercially produced Xylitol are birch trees and corncobs. In the form that comes from corn, the grain of the corn is never used. However, people sensitive to corn might look to other forms of Xylitol or use stevia instead. Note: Xylitol is typically sweeter than stevia; therefore, less Xylitol is needed when you would otherwise use sugar or stevia.

THE BAD

Agave Nectar, Honey and Maple Syrup

While it is true that these syrups are far less processed than white sugar, come from natural sources, and may even be organic, they are purely sugar at the molecular level and will cause a rise in blood sugar, insulin, and the body's inflammatory response. However, raw and organic forms of these syrups are far more identifiable and usable by the body than alternatives, which are highly refined, or created in a laboratory, and have no chance of being broken down safely.

While Maximized Living is not about "counting calories," we should acknowledge that these sweeteners will add unnecessary calories to your food or beverage, when the non-calorie sweeteners stevia and Xylitol are perfect replacements. When it comes to adding additional carbohydrates to your diet, particularly these simple sugars, keep in mind that the most dangerous carbohydrates for your health are the ones that are never used. So, use them sparingly, preferably on days of greatest activity or exercise.

THE UGLY

Artificial Sweeteners

While stevia and Xylitol come from earthly plants, artificial sweeteners come from manufacturing plants – which should be your first reason to doubt their claims of health benefits and/or safety.

Aspartame

This chemical has been used as a sugar substitute in diet soda since the 1980s. There are more than ninety-two different health side effects associated with aspartame consumption, including brain tumors, birth defects, diabetes, emotional disorders, and epileptic seizures. When aspartame is stored for long periods of time, or kept in warm areas, it changes to methanol, an alcohol that converts to formaldehyde and formic acid – known carcinogens. Although there are class-action lawsuits against aspartame underway throughout the country, it is well protected by the FDA and remains on the market today.

Splenda®

Splenda® has rapidly taken over the artificial sweetener market with claims that it is more natural because it comes from sugar. While that may be true, it takes several dozen chemical reactions in which sugar is chlorinated in order to become sucralose, the chemical name for Splenda®. This process involves chemically changing the structure of the sugar molecules by substituting three chlorine atoms for three hydroxyl groups. While chlorine is a known contaminant, further concerns are raised by the lack of studies on Splenda®. Aspartame has been studied thirty times more frequently to reveal its dangers. Few studies have been done on the short- and long-term effects of Splenda® or sucralose. With natural, non-manufactured products such as stevia so readily available, why wait for the studies?

Chapter 4

The Advanced Plan 🔱

Some individuals will require a more Advanced Plan to restore health and healing to their bodies. This plan may be used for short-term management of weight, disease, or detoxification, or may be used on a long-term basis for those who are genetically suited for it. The Advanced Plan has been researched and formulated to maximize your body's full potential for health, energy, recovery, and cognitive power. The Advanced Plan is designed to reduce inflammation, restore cell membrane function in order to aid detoxification, regulate hormones, and promote the use of fat as the body's primary source of energy.

Indications you may need this plan:

High triglycerides	Autism Spectrum Disorders
High cholesterol	Cancer
High blood pressure	Chronic fatigue
High blood sugar	Fibromyalgia
Low blood sugar	Heart disease
High insulin	Digestive dysfunction
High leptin	Obesity
Toxicity	Genetically intolerant to grains
Inflammatory disease	ADD/ADHD

There are many others who will benefit from the Advanced Plan. Those listed above absolutely need it.

The Advanced Plan may at first appear extreme. However, it is actually the easier meal plan to follow because it is designed to completely eliminate cravings. This is something several generations of low-calorie and low-fat diets have been unable to achieve, so it should come as no surprise that this plan is noticeably and fundamentally different from others you may have experienced.

THREE RULES ON THE ADVANCED PLAN

Fat	Protein	Carbohydrates
Increase your intake of healthy fats.	Moderate your intake of protein.	Eliminate grains, sugars and fruits.

Food Choices on the Advanced Plan

Follow the Three Principles of the Core Plan with the following modifications: Eliminate not only sugar but all foods that turn into sugar. These include:

 Grains
Even healthy grains rapidly convert to sugar and cause inflammation.

Most Fruits
Berries and Granny Smith apples are exceptions because they have a lower glycemic index and do not raise blood sugar levels as much as other fruits.

Excess Protein
Too much protein also will convert into sugar.

(If you need to lose weight, but are having difficulty succeeding on the Advanced Plan, reduce your protein intake first. On average, men should consume 20 grams of protein and women should consume 15 grams of protein per meal. Consume 5-10 additional grams of protein after exercise.)

Note: Removing all grains and sugars is easiest when they are removed completely and simultaneously. Although the first ten to fourteen days may be difficult, your body will adapt quickly, and cravings will be eliminated. Because the purpose of the Advanced Plan is to regulate hormones — not reduce calories — in order to be the most successful, removing grains and sugars cannot be started "gradually."

Over the first two to three weeks, while immediately eliminating all grains, sugars, and fruit, you should slowly increase your intake of good fats, because it is during this period that your body will be learning to burn fat as its primary fuel.

Carbohydrates to Eliminate on the Advanced Plan

Grains			
Barley	Brown Rice	Buckwheat	Bulgar (tabouli)
Millet	Rye	Semolina	Steel Cut Oats
Tapioca	Whole Grain Breads	Whole Grain Cereals	Whole Grains
Wheat Crackers	Ezekiel 4:9® Bread	Whole Grain Tortillas	

Root Vegetables and Tubers		
☒ Sweet Potato	☒ Yam	☒ Carrots

Fruit
Exceptions are berries, Granny Smith apples, lemons, limes, and avocados.

Carbohydrates to Moderate on the Advanced Plan

These carbohydrates may be consumed in small amounts on the Advanced Plan but not on a daily basis:

Artichokes	Leeks	Okra	Pumpkin
Tomatoes	Turnip	Legumes	Black Beans
Adzuki Beans	Black Beans	Chick Peas (garbanzo)	French Beans
Navy Beans	Kidney Beans	Lentils	Mung Beans
Yellow Beans	Pinto Beans	Split Peas	White Beans
Lima Beans	Squash (acorn, butternut, winter)		

Carbohydrates to Increase on the Advanced Plan

The Advanced Plan is NOT a "low-carb" diet. Be sure to replace the above lower-fiber and higher-glycemic carbohydrates with more of the high-fiber, low-glycemic carbohydrates below:

Arugula	Asparagus	Bamboo Shoots	Bean Sprouts
Beet Greens	Bell Peppers (red, yellow, green)	Broadbeans	Broccoli
Brussel Sprouts	Cabbage	Cassava	Cauliflower
Celery	Chayote Fruit	Chicory	Chives
Collard greens	Coriander	Cucumber	Dandelion Greens
Eggplant	Endive	Fennel	Garlic
Ginger Root	Green Beans	Hearts of Palm	Jicama (raw)
Jalapeno Peppers	Kale	Kohlrabi	Lettuce
Mushrooms	Mustard Greens	Onions	Parsley
Radishes	Radicchio	Snap Beans	Snow Peas
Shallots	Spinach	Spaghetti Squash	Summer Squash
Swiss Chard	Turnip Greens	Zucchini	Watercress

Why the Advanced Plan

No fruit? No grains?

At first glance, it might not seem realistic or even possible to eliminate grains, fruits, and sugars from your diet. After all, the USDA Food Pyramid suggests six to eleven servings of grains per day whether they are whole or refined. Canada's Food Guide has similar recommendations: five to twelve servings per day. And the guide mistakenly considers grains to be the foundation of a healthy diet.

Most people reading this book will realize that through the years, their diets have consisted largely of sugar, products that turn into sugar, and products with hidden sources of sugar. Therefore, at the cellular level, whether they realize it or not, most North Americans have been developing "Syndrome X," the metabolic syndrome that is a combination of medical disorders that include high blood pressure, obesity, high cholesterol, and diabetes. **Unfortunately, disease develops for years before it is finally diagnosed — and this dysfunction starts at the cellular level.**

Years of misguided meal plans will cause damaged cell membranes, which eventually leads to disease. The only way to reverse this trend is to follow the Advanced Plan, even for a period of time, to allow healing to take place at the cellular level.

The elimination of grains is not only necessary to reduce trauma to the cellular membrane, it is genetically a natural diet plan for many cultures. Our Paleolithic ancestors, specifically those from northern climates, hunted wild meats and gathered greens, vegetables, seeds, and berries. In reality, the human race has not changed much since that time, as described below by Loren Cordain, author of *The Paleo Diet*:

"DNA evidence shows that genetically, humans have hardly changed at all. To be specific, the human genotype has changed less than 0.02% in 40,000 years. This means that the genetic makeup of Paleolithic people is virtually identical to our own. Literally, we are Stone Agers living in the Space Age; our dietary needs are the same as theirs. Our genes are well adapted to a world in which all the food eaten daily had to be hunted, fished, or gathered from the natural environment - a world that no longer exists. Nature determined what our bodies needed thousands of years before civilization developed, before people started farming and raising domesticated livestock."

Dr. Boyd Eaton, published in the *New England Journal of Medicine*, writes:

"The foods we eat are usually divided into four basic groups. Two or more daily servings from each are now considered necessary for a balanced diet, but adults living before the development of agriculture and animal husbandry derived all their nutrients from two food groups. They apparently consumed cereal grains rarely, if at all."

So, the Advanced Plan takes us back not tens of thousands of years, but just a couple hundred. Historically, when a culture consumed 50 percent to 60 percent of its calories from grain, degenerative diseases rose proportionately.

> **The human race, and particularly northern cultures, has survived for tens of thousands of years without grains.**

We have done pretty well — until the last century.

The U.S. and Canadian food guides would have you believe that you can't get enough vitamins, minerals, and nutrients without fruits and grains, when this couldn't be further from the truth. Dr. Joel Fuhrman, author of *Eat to Live*, illustrates his classification of the nutrient densities in a variety of foods below (1,000 being a perfect score). While this reference does not take into consideration healthy fats and proteins needed for optimal well-being, it does illustrate that the highest ranking foods are vegetables, followed by fruits, and well ahead of grains. It would literally require eating **twenty bowls of oatmeal** to match the nutrients found in **one bowl of kale.**

Kale	1000	Tofu	86	Bananas	30
Collards	1000	Sweet Potatoes	83	Chicken Breast	27
Bok Choy	824	Apples	76	Eggs	27
Spinach	739	Peaches	73	Low Fat Yogurt, plain	26
Cabbage	481	Kidney Beans	71	Corn	25
Red Pepper	420	Green Peas	70	Almonds	25
Romaine Lettuce	389	Lentils	68	Whole Wheat Bread	25
Broccoli	342	Pineapple	64	Feta Cheese	21
Cauliflower	295	Avocado	64	Whole Milk	20
Green Peppers	258	Oatmeal	53	Ground Beef	20
Artichoke	244	Mangoes	51	White Pasta	18
Carrots	240	Cucumbers	50	White Bread	18
Asparagus	234	Soybeans	48	Peanut Butter	18
Strawberries	212	Sunflower Seeds	45	Apple Juice	16
Tomatoes	164	Brown Rice	41	Swiss Cheese	15
Plums	157	Salmon	39	Potato Chips	11
Blueberries	130	Shrimp	38	American Cheese	10
Iceberg Lettuce	110	Skim Milk	36	Vanilla Ice Cream	9
Orange	109	White Potatoes	31	French Fries	7
Cantaloupe	100	Grapes	31	Olive Oil	2
Flax Seeds	44	Walnuts	29	Cola	1

Teach Your Body to Burn Fat

Dr. Ron Rosedale explains:

"Health and life span is determined by the proportion of fat versus sugar people burn throughout their lifetime. The more fat you burn as fuel, the healthier you will be. The more sugar you burn as fuel, the more disease-ridden you will be, and the shorter your life will likely be."

While children may be capable of switching between primary fuel sources (sugar and fat), most adults have become full-time sugar burners due to a lack of healthy fats in the diet and by consuming an abundance of foods that turn into sugar. Thus, their body uses its immediate energy system (sugar) instead of its energy storage system (fat). The continual consumption of excess sugar, even healthy fruit and grain sugars, causes the body to store this sugar as fat unless it is needed for energy immediately. It doesn't take long before the body's fat-utilization system gets shut down completely.

Although grains and fruit aren't "manmade" foods, they do contain natural sugars and will break down into sugar once ingested. It is essential that sugar and anything that turns into sugar be eliminated on the Advanced Plan in order to fully restore the body's fat-burning mechanism and heal the cellular membranes. This includes grains and fruit.

Blood Pressure and Hormones

Insulin and Leptin

Central to the Advanced Plan is the rebalancing of the hormones insulin and leptin, which regulate cravings and the utilization of sugar vs. fat. Whether or not a person is overweight, it is vital to regulate these two superior hormones that control homeostasis, hunger, energy, and metabolism. Constant elevation of insulin, due to an abundance of sugar and grains in the diet, will cause a deficiency in the body's ability to store magnesium. That can lead to blood vessel constriction, elevated blood pressure, and coronary arterial spasms, which can result in a heart attack. Low magnesium interferes with the normal metabolism of essential fatty acids EPA and DHA, vital to the heart and brain.

Excess insulin also will create fluid retention. Many people with heart disease are advised to reduce their intake of salt (sodium), when it is the body's excess <u>retention</u> of sodium, caused by higher insulin and sugar levels, that elevates blood pressure and leads to congestive heart failure. Surprisingly, natural salt is a healthy source of twenty-one essential and thirty accessory minerals that are essential to your health. In contrast, refined table salt contains a much higher concentration of additives, including the true culprit: sugar.

Those who have become leptin-resistant, whose brains can no longer detect the presence of leptin, definitely need the Advanced Plan. The elimination of simple sugars, most fruits, and all grains that convert into sugar, is a vital step in allowing the body to re-establish normal leptin hormone cycles. That will help the body use fat, the primary source of fuel on the Advanced Plan. The Advanced Plan allows for the cellular insulin receptors to regenerate and for the leptin receptors in the brain to do the same.

Adaptation

When starting the Advanced Plan, realize that healthy fats typically have not been your primary source of fuel for years. Whether these fats are healthy or damaged, the body may have difficulty utilizing fat until it actually switches to fat-burning mode. For this reason, you should slowly incorporate more healthy fats over two to three weeks when starting the Advanced Plan. The elimination of sugar, grains and most fruits, however, must be done immediately and all at once. Even the smallest stimulation of sugar in the body will cause sugar cravings to persist.

Having been plagued by uncontrollable cravings for years, this adaptation period can be challenging for some. While many people will feel incredible the moment they eliminate inflammatory sugars, many will experience "withdrawal" symptoms similar to that of quitting smoking or coming off a powerful medication. When your body withdraws from sugar, symptoms of adaptation can be expected as your body may still have high insulin levels. These feelings may include fatigue, confusion, nausea, headaches, and general illness. Fortunately, the adaptation period typically lasts no longer than fourteen days. This time frame is dependent upon your body's natural cellular regeneration cycles.

Unfortunately, any indulgence in sugar during the adaptation period will interfere with hormone regulation — and set you back to Day 1. Therefore, removing all sugar immediately is truly the easiest way in the long run.

While one outcome of the Advanced Plan is the reduction of constant hunger and the need for constant snacking, you may require some healthy snacks during the first two weeks as insulin levels are adjusting. In fact, small snacks containing good fat and protein can help to stabilize insulin levels, which will help minimize any unpleasant symptoms during this transition.

Advanced Plan vs. Atkins®

North Americans have become aware of the dangers of fad diets, including the low-carbohydrate craze primarily fueled by the Atkins® Diet. One of the dangers of total restriction of carbohydrates from the diet is ketosis, an unhealthy state in which the body's liver begins to convert fat into fatty acids and ketone bodies and protein into nitrogenous waste in the blood stream. As the body works to expel this waste, serious damage may occur in the kidneys and liver. For that reason, even the low-carbohydrate diets do not advocate going into ketosis longer than fourteen days at a time.

In contrast, Maximized Living does not advocate you put your body into an abnormal state at all. Neither the Core nor Advanced Plan calls for a reduction of carbohydrates below your body's critical level. Both plans are **moderate-carbohydrate to high-carbohydrate diets** (not "low-carb"). Both plans are specifically **low sugar**. Be sure to get a substantial serving of carbohydrates with each meal but get them from lower-glycemic sources. In the Advanced Plan, get your carbohydrates from the best and most nutrient-rich source of all: vegetables.

Standard North American Diet	Low-Carb Craze	Maximized Living Core Plan	Maximized Living Advanced Plan
High Sugar (all sugar)	No Sugar (any sugar)	No Sugar (refined sugar)	No Sugar (anything that quickly forms sugar)
High Carb (bad carbs)	Low-Carb (bad and good carbs)	Moderate-to-High Carb (great carbs)	Moderate Carb (lowest-glycemic carbs)
Average Fat (low good fat, high bad fat)	High Fat (any fat)	Moderate Fat (good fat)	High Fat (good fat)
Moderate Protein (bad protein)	High Protein (any protein)	Moderate Protein (good protein)	Moderate Protein (good protein)

Time Frame on the Advanced Plan

Once you reach your health and wellness goals, (weight, blood sugar, cholesterol, symptoms, etc.), you may slowly re-introduce the healthy fruits and grains on the Core Plan. See how you respond with one serving of fruit and/or grains each day, and be sure to add only one food at a time. Your body's response will let you know quickly whether or not you need to remain on the Advanced Plan. *You also can verify your body's metabolic response through blood work, measuring blood pressure, etc.*

Notes
Toxicity and Weight-Loss Resistance – If you are not meeting your goals on the Advanced Plan and have already reduced your protein intake, you must consider toxicity as a cause of hormone disregulation and/or ongoing inflammation. Leptin levels are not only altered by the Standard North American Diet but also by toxins in our environment and food. **If toxicity is preventing you from reaching your goals, you may require a more advanced evaluation.** While the Advanced Plan alone will assist your body's ability to detoxify through the addition of healthy fats, and likely reduce toxicity-related symptoms by 30 percent to 50 percent, you may ask your Maximized Living provider about toxicity testing and/or cellular detoxification programs to help you reach your goals in conjunction with your Maximized Living Nutrition Plans.

Notes
Genetic Tendencies – Genetically, some people do better without ever consuming grains. In fact, there are many countries in the world where fruits and grains grow sparingly. Therefore, your genetic type must be taken into consideration when determining whether you need to stay on the Core or Advanced Plan once you reach your goals. Many people, particularly those with northern backgrounds, may prefer to stay on the Advanced Plan permanently.

Chapter 5

Why Are These Plans Different?

Many look at the Maximized Living Nutrition Plans and are surprised at how simple it is — no calories to count, no scales on the kitchen counter to weigh your portion sizes, no herbal supplements to manipulate your metabolism, and no packaged foods to order from the company headquarters. You can eat when you are hungry — just eat the right things. You trust your body's cues, not the clock, to tell you when it's time to eat.

Truthfully however, many others will have read the Plan and will already have lost sleep over how they will revamp the shopping list, what foods they will bring to work, and how on earth they will "survive" without sugar. (The truth is, sugar is an anti-nutrient, so you will survive much better without it). We realize that the Plan may not be easy at first, but it is simple in its guidelines. Like any other changes, lifestyle adjustments will take some time and planning ahead. But you will soon be back to quick trips "in and out" of the grocery store in no time. You may just be leaving with different things.

The Maximized Living Nutrition Plans is not a "diet" by the traditional definition, which implies restriction, deprivation, pain, and unsustainability. It is a nutrition plan for life. You will eat until you are full, you will likely stay full a lot longer, and you will naturally achieve results that you may not even see or understand. Both the Core and Advanced Plans adhere to the principle that there are foods that have been put on this planet specifically for us to eat. The closer the food is to its natural source, the better. The more altered by man, the worse. If weight loss is your goal, you can be assured that you will not only lose weight by eating this way, but you will be gaining health in the process. Many of the fad diets and traditional diet plans out there merely cause people to lose weight. Yet by eating processed and artificial foods, people put stress on their health. Why die young, just lighter?

Most other diet plans have some degree of compromise. Much of the focus on "how can I eat the foods I love and still lose weight?" has given birth to point systems, the development of artificial sweeteners, and "allowable" amounts of foods that are proven to damage your body. Your body knows the truth, and there is really no way to cheat the system. That doesn't mean that you will stick to the Maximized Living Plan 100 percent of the time. But when you get off track for a day or two, consider it a "vacation," and get back to basics quickly. Maximized Living is a way of life and something you can sustain over your lifetime — not just until you fit into a new pair of jeans.

Let's take a look at how it compares to some of the other popular diets out there.

Low-Carbohydrate Diets

Examples: Atkins™, South Beach®, The Zone Diet™

What's good:
These diets do a fairly good job at restricting bad carbohydrates, such as pretzels, chips, breads, pastas, and sugar.

What's bad:
These diets cater to the "sweet factor" by incorporating artificial sweeteners, such as aspartame, which turns into wood alcohol in the brain, and Splenda®, which starts as sugar but is chlorinated to make the finished product. See the special section on artificial sweeteners on page 48. Unfortunately, Purdue University research has shown that the regular use of artificial sweeteners may disrupt the body's natural ability to monitor caloric intake based on food sweetness, fundamentally shutting down the "satisfaction" trigger in the brain. This causes more hunger and more obesity. (Sources related to this topic are:
• *http://tinyurl.com/2mjbp*   • *http://tinyurl.com/l6yy7l*)

These diets don't differentiate between good fats and bad fats. That's why a cheesy, pork-filled, deluxe pizza may be acceptable on these diets, as long as you go easy on the crust. The restriction of bad carbohydrates shouldn't be countered with the over consumption of bad fats or other questionable foods that are "allowed," such as shellfish, cured meats, and manmade oils like margarine.

Low-Fat, Low-Calorie Diets

The low-fat diet craze has been in full swing since the early 1980s. We have been conditioned to think that fat is the enemy and that "low fat" is good.

What's Good
Low-calorie diets reduce the intake of sugar and encourage people to eat more vegetables.

What's Bad
Fat is the number one missing ingredient in the North American diet. This has contributed to a whole host of hormone problems and cognitive disorders, because these functions rely on fat as their metabolic building blocks. Low-fat diets reduce all fats, not just the bad fats.

More low-fat recommendations include:

- Fat-free salad dressings (usually loaded with sugar and/or vegetable oil)
- Reduced-fat dairy products (more processing and a higher percentage of sugar)
- Soy products (see page 40)
- Artificial sweeteners (see page 48)
- Restriction of eggs and all red meats, even healthy, grass-fed meats.

The Reality

North Americans eat more low-fat and low-calorie foods than any other part of the world, and yet we have the highest rates of obesity.

It is true that one gram of fat contains more calories than a gram of protein or carbohydrate. This is not to be feared but to be utilized. It means that fat is actually your body's preferred fuel for energy. We've been taught to avoid it because of its caloric density, when in fact we must realize that because of its caloric density it is most useful by the body for energy and satiety, provided your hormones are in order. (Consider the Advanced Plan if your fat-burning hormones are deregulated.)

Balanced Food Diets

Examples: The Zone™, Body for Life™

What's Good

These systems promote a moderation of protein, fat, and carbohydrates to maintain healthy insulin and leptin levels in the body.

What's Bad

There is very little differentiation between bad fats and good fats, healthy protein and unhealthy protein, and sugar may still be "acceptable" in certain quantities - even in their own packaged foods. While it's possible there is an ideal ratio of grain-fed meat to vegetable oil, these are not ideal or acceptable foods for your system when it comes to preventing disease.

Weight-Loss Systems and Clinics

Examples: Nutrisystem®, Jenny Craig®, Weight Watchers®

Through the years, these programs have helped thousands of people reach their weight-loss goals but have made no claims about reaching optimal health. While the North American weight-loss industry is clearly booming, so is disease in many thin people. We know we can do better. In Maximized Living, we don't want to see you spend your years counting points, only to "die lighter."

Typical "weight loss" snack:

INGREDIENTS: SOY NUGGETS (SOY PROTIN ISOLATE, OAT FLOUR, CALCIUM CARBONATE), GLYCERINE, POLY-DEXTROSE, HYDROLYZED COLLAGEN, CHOCOLATE CHIPS (MALTITOL, CHOCOLATE LIQUOR (PROCESSED WITH ALKALI), COCOA BUTTER, SOY LECITHIN, VANILLA EXTRACT), ROLLED OATS, PALM KERNEL AND PALM OIL, SUNFLOWER OIL, WHEY PROTEIN ISOLATE, COCOA POWDER (PROCESSED WITH ALALI), SOY NUTS, ROASTED ALMONDS, COCONUT, NATURAL AND ARTIFICIAL FLAVORS, WHOLE MILK POWDER, CELLULOSE, SOY LECI-THIN, SALT, SUCRALOSE, ACESULFAME, POTASSIUM AND VITAMIN MINERAL MIX (TRICALCIUM PHOSPHATE, CALCIUM CARBONATE, MAGNESIUM OXIDE, VITAMIN A PALMITATE, ASCORBIC ACID, SODIUM ASCORBATE, THIAMINE MONONITRATE, RIBOFLAVIN, PYRIDOXINE HYDROCHLORIDE, CYANOCABALAMIN, D-L ALPHA TO-COPHERYL ACTATE, NIACINAMIDE, BIOTIN, D-CALCIUM PANTOTHENATE, ZINC OXIDE, FOLIC ACID, CHROMIUM CHELATE, PHYTONADIONE, SODIUM SELENITE).

CONTAINS: SOY, MILK, TREE NUTS, WHEAT AND SULPHITES.

Beware of nutrition programs that rely heavily upon their own brands of snack bars and supplements. This "healthy" meal replacement bar from a popular international weight loss company isloaded with soy, damaged fats, and artificial sweeteners including sucralose. Unfortunately, the additional vitamins fortified into the product don't make up for the questionable foods that precede them on the ingredients list.

What's Good
These programs typically consider vegetables to be "all you can eat" or "free food." They also help people attain incredible results through accountability and weekly check-ins.

What's Bad
These programs typically rely on "point systems" for counting your portion sizes, calories, and food choices for the day. Unfortunately, point systems make little or no differentiation between quality foods versus chemical foods. If you use up too many points on a chocolate sundae, you're done for the day. In Maximized Living, we would rather see you add some healthy "points" to the "chocolate sundae" points so you actually get some nutrients to fuel your body. Point systems allow for many foods we know fuel diabetes, heart disease, and cancer when consumed in excess. What do these foods do in moderation?

Secondly, these types of programs rely heavily on the sales of their products that have questionable health benefits (see page 71, "reading labels.") It's not too difficult to understand that mail-order and boxed food that does not need to be refrigerated must contain unhealthy preservatives. It's time to get REAL (literally).

These programs have an incredible market share, so beware of celebrity endorsements. If even the spokespeople for these programs cannot commit to a long-term plan to keep their weight and health under control — and they are being paid to do it — you've got to wonder if you will succeed.

Vitamin Supplementation and Herbal Programs

What's Good
These programs, often developed by healthcare professionals, go beyond calorie counting to address the molecular science of one's body chemistry. There is typically a push for herbs, vitamins, and supplements that are more natural than low-calorie and nutrient-deficient foods.

What's Bad
Although Maximized Living endorses the use of the proper vitamins and supplements for each individual's needs, there are a few things to consider:

1) If your body is not well, you will not absorb the nutrients you need. That's where the five essentials of Maximized Living play a role, by addressing toxicity, the nerve system, exercise, and a healthy mind in conjunction with the foods you eat and supplements you take.

2) Supplements were designed to do just that: supplement one's diet. Vitamins and supplements taken without healthy fats, or not in the proper nutrient synergy because they have been extracted from their sources, have limited use in the

body. In Maximized Living we see people reach their optimal health by eating the food we were designed to eat in its original form — not once it's been through the laboratory. This will save you money, too.

3) Even if herbs and vitamins are taken properly, in conjunction with the appropriate foods, we acknowledge that not all people have the same body chemistry and therefore require unique diets. Without an Advanced Plan for those who need it, herbs will be a supplementary expense, not benefit.

For further information about proper ways to utilize vitamins and supplements, refer to Chapter 12.

Vegetarian and Natural Diets

Examples: Diet for a New America™ and the Rave Diet™

What's Good
Through recent years, North America has been waking up to the appalling realities of processed food and commercial meat.

What's Bad
Let's not forget that many cultures throughout history have survived on animal products without developing cancer and heart disease. It's important to note that these cultures have survived on natural meats and animal products, not the commercial animal products that are available today at the local grocery store. What has been a large source of confusion to the general public is that all studies linking heart disease and cancer to the consumption of animal products have been studying the wrong meats. Or they studied the disease in the wrong animals, such as rabbits, which are herbivores and not designed to eat meat at all.

Another deficiency is their oversight of genetic differences. New vegetarians often get put on high starchy carbohydrate diets when according to their genetic background they should naturally be eating lean meats, nuts, seeds, legumes and vegetables. While vegetarianism can certainly be a healthy way of living in many cultures, most North Americans attempting to eat this way become "grain-a-tarians" or "pasta-holics," which is not how true cultural vegetarians live.

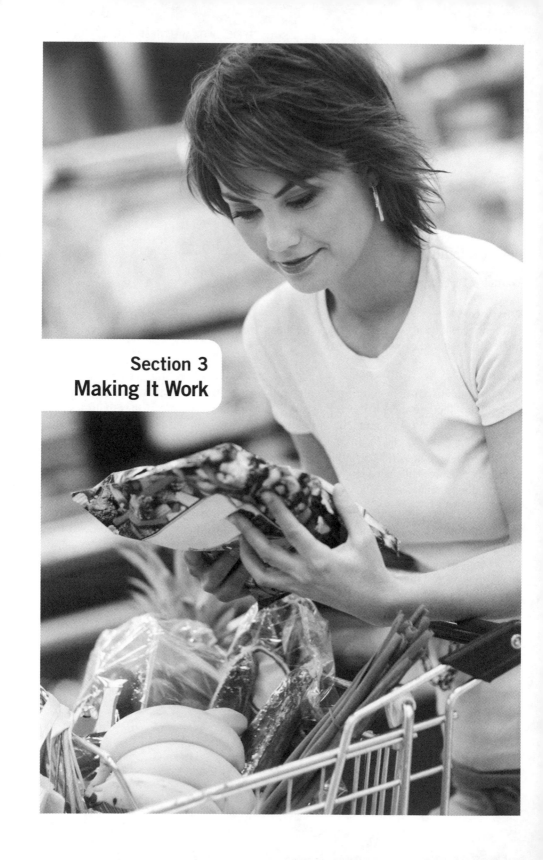

Section 3
Making It Work

Chapter 6

Meal Ideas
Core and Advanced Plans

Meal-Planning Tips

Consume Protein with Your Breakfast
- Higher protein meals increase your metabolism, suppress hunger later in the day, and stabilize leptin and blood sugar.

- Protein at breakfast is vital to increase your body's metabolic rhythm for the day — up to 30 percent for as long as twelve hours. (It's the equivalent of a 2-3 mile jog.)

- Many of us have grown up training our bodies to sustain energy on higher carbohydrate breakfasts. Particularly after the age of 40, and once leptin resistance becomes a problem, higher sugar meals and drinks in the morning are bound to create leptin problems later in the day.

- Hemp seeds, almond butter, whey protein, eggs, and healthy cheeses can be added to good fat and moderate carbohydrate breakfasts to ensure a decent serving of protein to start your day off right.

- Note: Since protein <u>activates</u> your metabolism, avoid having too much of it at dinner, as this can interfere with falling asleep. Excess protein (greater than 15-20 grams per female or 20-25 grams per male) will convert to sugar, creating further problems through the night and prevent fat burning from occurring.

Consume Fat With Every Meal
- Good fats play a vital role in hormone production, cancer prevention, regulation of metabolism, fat burning, brain development, and cellular healing by reducing inflammation.

- When your body has forgotten how to burn fat, the only way to retrain it is to give it the fuel it needs to burn. Lower-fat meals, high in carbohydrates, sugar, and protein, will forever keep your body out of a fat-burning state.

> **Leptin aka "The Fat-Burning Hormone"**
> Leptin is produced by your fat cells and is delivered to the brain's hypothalamus to regulate fat burning, hunger, cravings, and the sense of being full. Leptin sets up the body's repair mechanism through a cascade of hormones, which follow leptin. When leptin levels are in balance, you will lose weight easily on the Core Plan or just about any diet. Follow the recommendations in this chapter for optimum results.

Eat Slowly

- It takes approximately twenty minutes for your body's full signal to reach your brain. Eat slowly, push your plate aside when you are 80 percent finished, and allow your "full" signal to come on before you are overstuffed.

Leptin Resistance

When there is too much leptin being produced due to Standard North American Diet patterns and/or toxicity, the receptor sites on the brain's hypothalamus that detect leptin will actually burn out. When leptin can no longer be "heard" by the brain, leptin resistance develops and is the ultimate metabolic cause of one's inability to lose weight on any diet. It is the reason weight loss plateaus after initial success. This phenomenon also is called Weight-Loss Resistance. Those who are leptin-resistant should follow the Advanced Plan in Chapter 4 to re-establish leptin levels in the body. Leptin resistance also causes high glucose, insulin, and triglycerides in the blood. The constant snacking on empty and chemical-laden calories will prevent this fat-burning hormone from ever functioning in a normal rhythm as it would have in "hunter-gatherer" times.

Eat When You Are Hungry — Not Out of Habit

- Leptin was created to help you know when you are hungry and to regulate fat burning in the absence of food or sugar.

- Therefore, Maximized Living endorses eating when you are hungry — not counting calories or timing a certain number of meals each day. When your system is free of nerve interference, toxic interference, and/or dietary stress, you will be able to sense when and how much you need to eat.

- When you are eating enough good fat, you will remain full for several hours. When you are eating too many high-starch, high-glycemic, low-fiber carbohydrates, you will be continuously hungry. Be sure to eat enough fat and as few starchy carbohydrates as possible to prolong your feeling of fullness.

- Once your hormone levels are normalized, a healthy meal should last you five hours between daytime meals. While snacking is traditionally thought to boost your metabolism, it actually alters the normal operations of your hormones, which ultimately control your metabolism. Our evolutionary mechanisms were designed to deal with periods of starvation, not constant snacking, which raises triglycerides and insulin in the blood and impedes the entrance of leptin into the brain to control hunger and fat burning.

- If you must snack:

    - Be sure to consume a snack with as much fat, protein, and fiber as possible. (Nuts are great.) Do NOT snack on starchy carbohydrates. Regardless of how many or how few carbohydrates you eat for a snack, the change in insulin levels will create hunger again within a short period of time.

    - Evaluate what you ate at your last full meal so you do not repeat the same mistake.

Avoid Eating after Dinner

- The fat-burning hormone leptin works on a 24-hour rhythm. Overnight, it coordinates the body's repair systems, which include melatonin, thyroid hormone, growth hormone, sex hormones, and the immune system.

- Your body repairs itself during sleep while burning fat, provided leptin is in balance. When leptin is within normal range, the body's prime hours of fat burning occur in the final three to four hours of overnight sleep. Healthy leptin levels would naturally increase at night and be received by the brain to slow down the cravings, reduce hunger, and accelerate the burning of fat for energy through the night. If your leptin is out of balance, eating after dinner will alter your body's attempts to stabilize it.

- If your leptin is normal, nighttime snacks will eventually cause leptin to become deregulated, because late meals cause leptin to swing in the opposite direction.

Starting on a new program can be confusing and overwhelming at first, so here is a sample seven-day menu plan to help you get started. This is meant to be a guide. You can customize your meal plan to suit your own needs and taste. These are simple, straightforward, and do not require a recipe. However, we encourage you to use the recipe section in this book to add more variety and zest to your meals.

Core Plan Menu Ideas

	Breakfast	Lunch	Snack	Dinner
Day 1	Smoothie	Tomato Soup with Not Tuna Salad	Whole Grain Tortillas with Salsa and Guacamole	Cole Slaw with Roasted Vegetables and ¼ cup of Hemp Seeds
Day 2	Eggs with Whole Grain Toast	Leftover Chicken with Quinoa and Spinach Salad	Crackers and Veggies with Hummus	Grilled Steak with No-tatoes and Green Beans
Day 3	Smoothie	Chili over Brown Rice with Spinach	Trail Mix (mixture of raw nuts and seeds)	Chicken Salad on Greens with Almonds
Day 4	Oatmeal with Sliced Banana and Nuts	Taco Salad on Brown Rice and Greens (Using Leftover Chili)	Whole Grain Crackers with Cheese and Olives	Bison Burgers with Steamed Broccoli on Salad
Day 5	Smoothie	Turkey Reuben Sandwich	Celery with Baba Ganoush or Tahini Dip	Greek Salad with Grilled Chicken
Day 6	Eggs, Any Style over Spinach	Hemp Seed Salad with Stuffed Portobello Mushroom	Almond Power Bar	Salmon with Asparagus and Roasted Cauliflower
Day 7	Yogurt with Fruit	Veggie Wrap w/ Hummus Spread	Chocolate Bark with Nut Butter or Raw Nuts	Curry Chicken with Broccoli and Field Greens Salad

Advanced Plan Menu Ideas

When following the Advanced Plan menu, it's important to include some high-quality fats (i.e. olive oil, butter, hemp seed oil, flax meal, olives, avocados, raw nuts, seeds, coconut, full-fat organic dairy, etc.) plus a moderate amount of protein (15 grams for women and 25 grams for men) with each meal. This will keep you feeling satisfied for several hours.

	Breakfast	Lunch	Snack	Dinner
Day 1	Smoothie	Greek Salad with Turkey Burger	Raw Nuts and Sea Salt Trail Mix	Chicken Breast with Oven Roasted Vegetables
Day 2	Veggie Omelette with or without Cheese	Cole Slaw and Hemp Seeds in Salad	Almond Power Bar	Grilled Beef Steak with Green Beans and Roasted Tomatoes
Day 3	Yogurt and Berries (with or without added Whey Protein)	Chicken Salad on Greens with Almonds	Granny Smith Apple with Almond Butter, Cinnamon and Pumpkin Seeds	Cabbage Salad with Hemp Seeds
Day 4	Baked Granny Smith Apple with Cinnamon & Stevia plus two eggs	Buffalo Chicken Wraps (Chicken, Hot Sauce, Blue Cheese in Lettuce)	Chopped Coconut or Coconut Flakes	Mini Grass-Fed Burgers with Roasted Cauliflower
Day 5	Smoothie	Chicken Caesar Salad	Red Peppers and Tahini Dip	Fancy Salmon over Greens with Sauteed Zucchini
Day 6	Artichoke Fritatta	Leftover Salmon on Greens	Baba Ganoush and Celery	Fish Fry with Steamed Vegetables and Salad
Day 7	Green Smoothie	Ground Turkey Zucchini Boats	Raw Veggies and Hummus	Grilled Lamb with Roasted Eggplant and Greek Salad

Special Focus: Beverages and Water

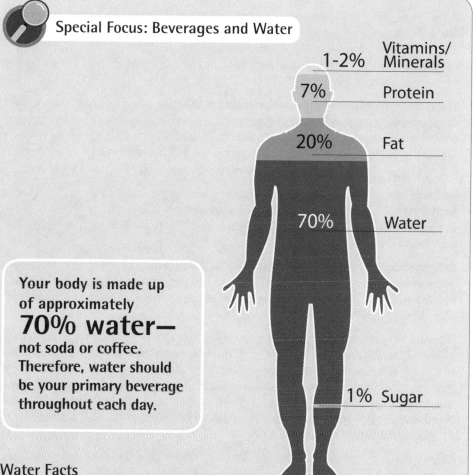

1-2% Vitamins/Minerals

7% Protein

20% Fat

70% Water

1% Sugar

Your body is made up of approximately 70% water— not soda or coffee. **Therefore, water should be your primary beverage throughout each day.**

Water Facts

• Lack of water is the number one trigger of daytime fatigue.

• Your body loses as much water when you are asleep as when you are awake.

• Your body needs as much water in cold weather as it does in warm weather.

• Research indicates that eight to ten glasses of water a day could significantly ease back and joint pain for up to 80 percent of sufferers.

• A mere 2 percent drop in body water can trigger brain fog and short term memory impedance.

• Drinking five glasses of water daily decreases the risk of colon cancer by 45 percent, breast cancer by 79 percent, and bladder cancer by 50 percent.

Most North Americans understand the importance of drinking more water, yet 98 percent remain chronically dehydrated. Your body needs a minimum of 50 ounces of water per 100 ounces of body weight per day. A person weighing 150 pounds would therefore need 2 quarts of water per day — that's slightly larger than a 2-liter bottle.

At the same time, North Americans realize that there are varying qualities of drinking water. Twenty years ago bottled water was unheard of. Today, consumption of bottled water increases every year. Rightfully, many people are starting to question whether bottled or "healthy" water is at all necessary, just a fad, or any better than water out of the tap.

While all North American cities must meet strict drinking water standards with respect to cleanliness, these standards are primarily related to concentrations of microorganisms, organic compounds, raw sediment, and large concentrations of inorganic compounds in the water. Thanks to these practices of hygiene, we don't have the water contamination hazards they do in countries around the world where water-borne illnesses are rampant.

However, today we face a new challenge: The very chemicals that are used in water treatment facilities to protect us from microorganisms are ironically linked to more dangerous diseases. Nearly all cities in North America treat their water with chlorine and fluoride, which pose health hazards of their own.

Chlorine may kill microbes, but it reacts with organic compounds that occur naturally in water to form chlorination byproducts (CBP's). Some CBP's have been flagged by the FDA as known carcinogens, and others are known to cause cell and genetic mutation and oxidation of cholesterol. *(Epidemiology.)*

Fluoride has been touted to prevent tooth decay, despite years of research and recognition by the FDA that such is not the case. You may recall receiving fluoride treatments as a child, or your children may be receiving them now. Even your dentist knows that fluoride should not be swallowed. Because fluoride, when ingested, is known to cause serious health problems, including tissue breakdown, bone weakness, cancer, and auto-immune diseases, it has been banned in a number of European countries. (Curnette, et al, *Journal of Clinical Investigation.)*

Medications – While not added to drinking water in water treatment facilities, concentrations of medications flushed down the toilet or passed through a person's urine have been detected in cities across North America. Everything, from birth control pills to antidepressants, has been shown to bypass the city's water filtration system, ending up in your home and your body. The side-effects from medications are far too numerous to list. By drinking city water, you may be popping pills without even knowing it. (Donn, et al, *Associated Press.)*

Lead and other heavy metals, which are known neurotoxins, are an additional problem cropping up in cities across the continent. Because neighborhood pipes and infrastructure may not be subject to the same standards as the city's water treatment facilities, the leaching of heavy metals into water that reaches your home may occur even if your municipality is meeting its citywide standards. (Sher, *Sun Media.)*

Does that mean we all need to drink bottled water?
There are as many people concerned about the environmental hazards of plastic bottles as there are people concerned about the toxicity of city water. Fortunately, you have a number of options:

Bottled Water

Without making any functional or structural changes to your home, you can opt for bottled water that is cleaner than all tap waters. Reverse Osmosis (RO) and distilled bottled water are more reliable for cleanliness than natural "spring" waters, because RO and distilled water go through a more stringent purification process. You can determine from the label whether there is chlorine or fluoride in the water.

If you do drink bottled water from plastic bottles, avoid having the plastics heat up in high summer temperatures or allowing them to thaw after they have been frozen. There are many in the water-filtration industry, who are concerned with leaching.

Carbon Filter Pitchers

Pitchers with carbon filters, such as the Brita® and PUR®, are another step in the right direction. Carbon faucet filters do the same job of filtering most inorganic compounds out of the water. Unfortunately, the pitcher filters have a minimal capacity to eliminate fluoride, chlorine and CBP's.

Faucet Carbon Filters

Individual carbon filters for your faucets must be changed regularly but are economical and remove most chlorine and fluoride. Unfortunately, CBP's are too small and cannot be filtered out or removed by faucet filters.

Reverse Osmosis (RO) Filters

An RO system, which sits under your sink, may use a great deal of water in the process of purifying it, but it will remove CBP's that are missed by carbon filters. While they are more costly, they may last longer and certainly are more effective.

Distillation

Distillation of water provides for even greater purity than does RO filtration. Like RO, it is a slow process and uses more water than you need. More cumbersome than RO, you will need a storage tank for the unit away from your sink. While distillation creates impeccably pure water, it becomes acidic from absorbing carbon dioxide from the air. So, you are better off removing toxins through filtration and allowing trace minerals to remain, rather than creating a super-pure form of water that does not occur in any stream on earth.

Note: Your greatest susceptibility to toxins in city water is not when you drink it, but when you shower or bathe in it. As your pores warm and open up, the intoxication occurs six times faster than when drinking the same water. In the shower, toxins can be absorbed by inhalation of vapors, in addition to the water being absorbed by your open pores. In a ten-minute shower, the body takes in more chlorine than it would if drinking eight glasses of the same water. *(Consumer Reports)* For this reason, carbon filters in the shower or whole-home filtration (below) should be considered.

House Filtration

Traditionally, these systems have cost tens of thousands of dollars. But recently, they have become much more affordable – often $1,000-$3,000. A house filtration system not only ensures safe drinking water but will save you the expense of installing and replacing filters on individual taps and showers throughout your home. It also prevents toxic chemicals and CBP's from getting into your dishwasher or laundry.

Chapter 7

The Grocery Store

Most people want to make nutritional improvements, but taking on the grocery store can be daunting. Shopping can be a challenge if you don't know or have the right information.

The emergence of organic foods has helped many people make better choices but has still left us with questionable items in our shopping carts. Low-carbohydrate beer and organic chocolate are classic examples. This section is designed to help you make the right choices on your Maximized Living Nutrition Plans.

Shopping Success Tips

Where to Shop
When buying organic, remember to start "at the top of the food chain," specifically with animal products. Not only are grocery stores carrying more natural and organic choices, but you can choose from health food stores, food co-ops, local farmers, and online resources for your organic products. When buying directly from the farmer, you might spend less for organic, grass-fed meat than you would in the grocery store for commercial meat.

To save money, refer to the "Pesticides in Produce" Wallet Guide from foodnews.org, which you can find on page 79. This guide shows which vegetables have the lowest pesticide load, which can be helpful when deciding to buy conventional vs. organic.

The majority of your food can be found right in the regular grocery store. Chances are you won't need the health food store or specialty items more often than every two to three weeks.

Build your own resource manual with the help of the shopping guide at the end of this chapter. Identify your favorite brands and where to purchase them for the best price.

Stocking Up
Keep a good stock of your basics at all times so you can pull together a "surprise meal" quickly without an emergency trip to the grocery store. (See page 81, "The Pantry.")

Schedule a weekly time for your grocery and health food store shopping. When it comes to food choices, emergency shopping usually encourages bad decisions. There should be regular replenishments of the good foods in your pantry, because the items at the back of your shelves are not typically the healthiest.

Make shorter and more regular visits to the store for fruit and vegetables every two to three days. You'll get the freshest produce and you won't lose money watching it spoil. Remember fruits and vegetables lose valuable nutrients the longer they sit, and conventional produce usually spends a long time in transit. The less time it stays in your kitchen, the better. Fresh is always best; frozen is next best, and canned is least desirable.

Keep your shopping list somewhere handy so it can be updated as you go through your week. Don't wait until Saturday morning to stare into your refrigerator or pantry thinking "What do we need this week?" Instead, as you run out of items, or think of something you need, keep your list nearby and up-to-date. You might want to use a separate list for each store you visit.

In the Store

Shop around the outside of the store where the good choices reside. When you get into the inner aisles of the store, you'll find more packaged, processed, and less healthy foods. (Compare the smaller European grocery stores, which have few aisles in contrast to our North American megastores. Adding more inner aisles to our stores hasn't been a good thing for our health.)

Write out your shopping list in the order that the store is arranged so that you can move systematically without having to back track.

Get to know the store and department managers where you shop. They are usually happy to help. If there is an item you prefer, ask if they can stock it. Sometimes they are willing to custom order items for you. Let them know what you would like to see in the store. For natural foods that may carry a slightly higher price tag, ask about discounts available when you stock up on larger quantities.

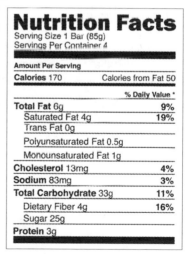

Reading Labels

Traditional diets have taught North Americans to become obsessed with reading food labels. But it's clear that our methods haven't worked well for most because we've been taught to read the wrong part of the label.

In Maximized Living, we know you will fill up — not on calories — but on nutrients. Therefore, the grams of fat, serving size, and any related points that may otherwise go along with foods you buy, are far less important than the ingredients. This is where you really need to be looking first.

What's Important

- Focus on the ingredients portion of the label.

- Look for a minimal number of ingredients — the less the better. You can dress it up once you buy it.

- Look for natural ingredients, such as the items included on the Core Plan. (Avoid ingredients you can't read or pronounce because they were probably made in a laboratory).

- Buy more foods that aren't required to have labels because what you see is what you get (i.e. fruits and vegetables).

- Make a habit of checking the label on each item you buy. It won't be long before you will know exactly what to consider. It will quickly become a habit and won't add any extra time to your trip to the store.

Typical Packaged Food Label

INGREDIENTS: WATER - SPRING WATER. SUGAR FREE STRAWBERRY GELATIN - ARTIFICIALLY FLAVORED - WATER, GELATIN, ADIPIC ACID (FOR TARTNESS), SODIUM CITRATE (CONTROLS ACIDITY), CITRIC ACID (FOR TARTNESS), ASPARTAME** AND ACESULFAME POTASSIUM (SWEETENERS), SALT, RED 40, ARTIFICIAL FLAVOR. **PHENYLKETONURICS: CONTAINS PHENYLALANINE. SUB BUN - ENRICHED BLEACHED WHEAT FLOUR ([WHEAT FLOUR, NIACIN, REDUCED IRON, THIAMIN MONONITRATE {VITAMIN B1}, RIBOFLAVIN {VITAMIN B2}, FOLIC ACID], MALTED BARLEY FLOUR), WATER, SUGAR, WHITE WHEAT BRAN, CONTAINS 2% OR LESS OF THE FOLLOWING: SOYBEAN OIL, YEAST, WHEAT GERM, DOUGH CONDITIONERS (MONO & DIGLYCERIDES, SODIUM STEAROYL LACTYLATE, ENZYME MODIFIED SOY LECITHIN, DATEM), SALT, GUAR GUM, MODIFIED CELLULOSE, CALCIUM PROPIONATE (PRESERVATIVE), XANTHAN GUM, ARTIFICIAL FLAVORS, ENZYMES. CONTAINS: WHEAT, SOY. COOKED HAM - WATER ADDED - CHOPPED AND FORMED - SMOKE FLAVOR ADDED - HAM, WATER, CONTAINS LESS THAN 2% OF SALT, POTASSIUM LACTATE, MODIFIED CORN STARCH, SODIUM LACTATE, SODIUM PHOSPHATES, SUGAR, SODIUM DIACETATE, SODIUM ASCORBATE, SODIUM NITRITE, NATURAL AND ARTIFICIAL FLAVOR, SMOKE FLAVOR. 2% MILK REDUCED FAT AMERICAN PASTEURIZED PREPARED CHEESE PRODUCT - PASTEURIZED PART-SKIM MILK, WATER, MILKFAT, MILK PROTEIN CONCENTRATE, SODIUM CITRATE, MILK, CONTAINS LESS THAT 2% OF LACTIC ACID, SORBIC ACID AS A PRESERVATIVE, SALT, WHEY PROTEIN CONCENTRATE, OLEORESIN PAPRIKA (COLOR), ANNATTO (COLOR), VITAMIN A PALMITATE, ENZYMES, CULTURE, CHEESE CULTURE WITH CORNSTARCH ADDED FOR SLICE SEPARATION. CONTAINS: MILK. CHOCOLATE CHIP COOKIES - UNBLEACHED ENRICHED FLOUR (WHEAT FLOUR, NIACIN, REDUCED IRON, THIAMINE MONONITRATE [VITAMIN B1], RIBOFLAVIN [VITAMIN B2], FOLIC ACID), SEMISWEET CHOCOLATE CHIPS (SUGAR, CHOCOLATE, COCOA BUTTER, DEXTROSE, SOY LECITHIN - AN EMULSIFIER, MILK), PALM OIL, HIGH FRUCTOSE CORN SYRUP, SUGAR, DEXTROSE, CORNSTARCH, SALT, BAKING

Common Mistakes

- Spend less time looking at grams of fat, carbohydrates, proteins, calories, and serving size. Remember that the "recommended daily values" on this part of the label do not take into consideration age, gender, athletic activity, or specific dietary needs.

- Beware of boisterous advertising claims. Cereals have recently been under the microscope by the FDA for claiming outrageous health benefits, such as "low in fat" or "trans-fat free," while clearly listing unhealthy, dangerous ingredients on the label. The advertisers want you to SEE "Low in Cholesterol," (which doesn't matter), and MISS "high-fructose corn syrup" on the ingredients list.

- Being low in fat, low in carbohydrates or sugar-free does not make something healthy.

- Being organic or located in the health food section of the store, (i.e. organic sugar or organic potato chips), does not make something good for you.

Watch Out for the Following Common Hidden Ingredients:

- Various forms of sugar (foods ending in "ose")

- Monosodium Glutamate (MSG), a powerful stimulator of free radical production in the body

- Hydrolyzed or autolyzed ingredients (highly heated, addictive excitotoxins)

- Artificial sweeteners (sucralose/Splenda®, aspartame/Nutrasweet®, Equal® among others)

- Hydrogenated or partially-hydrogenated oils. These trans fats may still appear on the ingredients list, but if the quantity per serving is less than 500 mg, the food can boast "trans-fat free" on the label. You may notice the serving size has conveniently "shrunk" over the years.

- Refined flour touted as "organic." If it isn't "sprouted, whole grain, or stone-ground" it is refined.

- Additives, colorings, chemicals, and preservatives.

Deli Meats and Seafood Counter

The deli counter can print out the ingredient label for anything you are ordering. The seafood counter typically will have a list of water sources for their fish. This information will help you make the right decision.

For the most part, deli meats are not healthy. However, if you are going to buy deli meats, stay away from MSG, nitrates, nitrites, artificial preservatives, and by-products. Many of the flavored and spiced lunchmeats contain additives and preservatives. Just like any other food item, the fewer ingredients, the better. Some organic brands are available now.

If you are like most people, your first few weeks of Maximized shopping may come as a shock. But rest assured, you will soon be at peace with your new way of life. The extra time in the grocery store during the first few weeks will pay off in your health and pocketbook very quickly. Although you may need to invest extra time getting started, it won't be long before you are "in and out" of the grocery store once again.

Shopping List

Fill in your favorite local brands and retailers for foods on the Maximized Living Nutrition Plans. Ask your Maximized Living Doctor for a customized directory for your region, or for products and supplements which may be available in the Maximized Living Health Center

Core = **O**   Advanced = **⬆**   Raw = **🌱**

	FOOD TYPE	LOCAL BRAND NAMES	LOCAL RETAILER/ SOURCE
	PROTEIN CHOICES		
O **⬆**	Cold-water fish		
	Wild Pacific or Alaskan is best.		
O **⬆**	Small Fish		
	Anchovies, sardines in olive oil		
O **⬆**	Eggs		
	Eggs from free-range, hormone and antibiotic-free chickens are better than eggs from caged and injected chickens fed organic foods or omega-3s		

	FOOD TYPE	LOCAL BRAND NAMES	LOCAL RETAILER/ SOURCE
◉ ⚱ ❧	Raw Cheeses		
	Most naturally occurring and healthiest form of cheese. (Beware of rice and soy alternatives.)		
◉ ⚱	Beef		
	100% grass-fed -- you must ask! Some farms grain feed the animals "at the end," which is still not desirable. This alters their vitamin E content and fatty acid ratios. Please note that "organic" does NOT mean grass-fed. Check with local farms, co-ops and online.		
◉ ⚱	Chicken		
	Free-range, hormone-free and antibiotic-free is best. "Free from antibiotics" and "naturally raised" are steps in the right direction.		
◉ ⚱	Turkey		
	Free-range, hormone- freeand antibiotic-free is best. Look for natural turkey "bacon" without nitrites or sugar.		
◉ ⚱ ❧	Whey Protein		
	Whey from raw mik and grass fed cows is best utilized and least harmful. (Most commercial brands are heated at high temperatures and may contain excitotoxins and/or artificial sweeteners).		
◉ ⚱ ❧	Protein Supplement / Complete Meal Replacement		
	Avoid commercial soy and whey products -- acceptable plant-based products should either be fermented soy, sprouted rice, or hemp-seed based.		
◉ ⚱	Egg Protein		
	Great for baking -- can also substitute for eggs or egg whites. If not available, use whey protein plus 1 egg (best and most similar tasting substitute)		
◉ ⚱ ❧	Shelled Hemp Seeds		
	Incredible protein source for salads and/or mixed with vegetables to produce a complete meal. w4 Tablespoons = 22 grams of protein		
	FAT CHOICES		
◉ ⚱ ❧	Raw Nuts and Seeds		
	Look for raw, consider organic. Often available raw at bulk food stores. Store in the refrigerator to maintain the integrity of the fats.		
◉ ⚱ ❧	Olive Oil, Olives, Grape Seed Oil		
	Extra virgin is best. extra virgin olive oil should be stored in a dark container to block the light.		

	FOOD TYPE	LOCAL BRAND NAMES	LOCAL RETAILER/ SOURCE
O ⚡ 🌱	Coconut Oil		
	Coconut oil is the ideal oil for cooking, baking, and frying, as it does not denature with high heat. Extra virgin is best, virgin or non-virgin is acceptable for greasing the pan.		
O ⚡	Coconut Flakes		
	Toasted flakes are delicious on salad or as a snack.		
O ⚡	Coconut Flour		
	Great alternative to grain flour for baking, thickening sauces, and great in smoothies.		
O ⚡ 🌱	Coconut Butter		
	Not for cooking, but for eating!		
O ⚡ 🌱	Coconut Milk		
	Full-fat coconut milk is thicker than watered down versions. This becomes a personal preference.		
⚡ ⚡ 🌱	Flax Seeds, Flax Seed Meal		
	Ground flax meal is great on salads, in oatmeal, and as a healthy substitute for flour in baking.		
O ⚡ 🌱	Flax Seed Oil, Cod Liver Oil		
	Do not heat!		
O ⚡ 🌱	Hemp Seed Oil		
	Best ratio of essential fatty acids — mix into salad dressings, smoothies, oatmeal — everything!		
O ⚡ 🌱	Fish Oil (supplement)		
	Look for fish oil that has been molecularly filtered to eliminate any contamination. Fish oil with essential fats in the 4:1 ratio is ideal.		
O ⚡	Nut Butters (almond, macadamia)		
	Raw is best but can be difficult to find.		
O ⚡	Tahini		
	Raw is best		
O ⚡	Yogurt		
	Full-fat, plain, organic. Raw is best, if available. No sugar!		

Core = O   Advanced = ⚡   Raw = 🌱

	FOOD TYPE	LOCAL BRAND NAMES	LOCAL RETAILER/ SOURCE
⊙ ⏚	Butter		
	Organic (raw is best, if available)		
⊙ ⏚	Milk		
	Full-fat, organic is a bare minimum. (Non-homogenized is even better. Non-pasteurized is best if available.)		
⊙⏚🌱	Chocolate (cocao)		
	Pure chocolate contains no sugar. Mix or melt down with stevia and/or cinnamon instead. Use in yogurt, smoothies, or with nuts/berries for a dessert or snack. Look for 100% chocolate squares (Baker's® Chocolate) or chocolate powder, sometimes available at bulk food stores.		
	HIGH-FIBER CARBOHYDRATE CHOICES		
⊙⏚🌱	Vegetables		
	Organic is best, but essential. Referto the EWG's "Dirty Dozen" and "Clean 15" on page 70 — Vegetables with the highest pesticide loads should be bought organic.		
⊙⏚🌱	Greens Drinks		
	Great substitute for essential vegetables if lacking in your diet — and great for children! Watch out for additives in commercial brands.		
	STARCHY CARBOHYDRATE CHOICES		
⊙⏚🌱	Starchy Vegetables		
	Organic is best, but not essential.		
⊙⏚🌱	Beans		
	Dried, in bulk or in bags (organic is best, but not essential.)		
⊙ ⏚	Canned Beans		
	No salt added is preferred.		
⊙ ⏚	Refried Beans		
	Flavored brands also available using healthy spices		
⊙	Whole Grains and Whole Cereals		
	Must be "whole grain, sprouted, or stone-ground."		

	FOOD TYPE	LOCAL BRAND NAMES	LOCAL RETAILER/ SOURCE
O	Whole Grain Breads, Bagels, English Muffins, etc.		
	Every grain ingredient on the label must read "whole grain, sprouted, or stone-ground." (Must freeze this type of bread).		
	CONDIMENTS, SPICES, AND SEASONINGS		
O	Mayonnaise		
	Most substitutes readily available in grocery stores (including some brands of mayo substitute Vegenaise®) are made with canola oil and/or soy products. Grapeseed oil and olive oil based spreads are acceptable.		
O	Salad Dressing		
	Most store brands use rancid oils — copy the ingredients and make your own healthy dressings with acceptable replacement ingredients! Hemp seed oil has the ideal 4:1 ratio of omega 3's and 6's.		
O	Tamari		
	Fermented soy product, excellent substitute for traditional soy or steak sauce.		
O	Marinades		
	Bragg's Liquid Amino's or Liquid Soy is a healthy form of soy - and great for meat.		
O	Herbs and Spices		
	Herbs in bulk are most economical. Organic spices are best (not irradiated). Look for individual "blends" (Greek Seasoning, Herbs of Provence and Salad Sprinkles) gomasio (sesame seeds with garlic, sea salt, and/or seaweed) - great on salads and vegetables.		
O	Salsa		
	Look for no-sugar salsa; organic is best.		
O	Tapenade		
	Also very easy to make at home		
O	Salt		
	The words "sea salt" aren't enough! General sea salt may still contain 2% additives, including sugar — check the labels! Some of the best, unrefined sea salts are Celtic Sea Salt and Himalayan Salt -- you will see flecks of color in the salt which shows that the minerals are unprocessed and intact.		

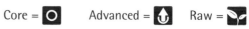

Core = **O**   Advanced = 🔱   Raw = 🌱

	FOOD TYPE	LOCAL BRAND NAMES	LOCAL RETAILER/ SOURCE
	SWEETENERS		
▣ 🔱 🍸	Stevia		
	Look for stevia without unnatural preservatives and additives. Brands come in a variety of tastes and concentrations.		
▣ 🔱	Xylitol		
	Some people prefer the taste of Xylitol over stevia. Be sure to use a Xylitol that does not contain additional corn-based additives.		

(Lerner, et al, *Maximized Living Makeover.*)

Produce

Most Americans have a preference as to the fruits and vegetables they like to eat. However, most people don't eat nearly enough vegetables and don't include enough variety. The typical go-to vegetables are iceberg lettuce, tomatoes, broccoli, and green beans. The first two (lettuce and tomatoes) are number one in the country only because they are used on most fast-food hamburgers. The last two (broccoli and beans) are often soaked in sauces, smothered with cheese, and overcooked. There are so many other vegetables available today that will help you increase your daily intake. Expand your horizons. Look especially for locally grown and in-season vegetables for maximum freshness and nutrients.

Remember: The most important and economical change, when it comes to organic food, is to start with purchasing organic animal products. Ideally, people should be eating a 100 percent organic, whole-food diet. As you expand your horizons and incorporate more fruits and vegetables into your diet, you may choose to go organic on these items as well. If cost is a concern, the following are the produce items that should be purchased organically because they have the heaviest pesticide load. This list is updated yearly by the Environmental Working Group and can be found at foodnews.org. This Web site will give you the full list of pesticide loads. But here are the top twelve "dirtiest" and fifteen "cleanest" fruits and vegetables most commonly found in today's market.

Every kitchen needs to be stocked with staple items so that meals can be prepared quickly and efficiently. If you enjoy preparing food and are already a cooking pro, you know that having the items readily available is very important. If you are just getting to know your kitchen better, this is where you must start — gathering the essentials.

Special Focus: Pesticides

The Environmental Working Group in Washington, D.C., has developed the Shopper's Guide to Pesticides based on data from nearly 87,000 tests for pesticide residues in produce between 2000-2007 and collected by the USDA and the FDA.

THE DIRTY DOZEN SHOULD BUY THESE ORGANICALLY (highest pesticide load)	THE CLEAN FIFTEEN OK TO BUY CONVENTIONAL (lowest pesticide load)
1. Peaches	1. Onion
2. Apples	2. Avocado
3. Bell Peppers	3. Sweet Corn
4. Celery	4. Pineapple
5. Nectarines	5. Mango
6. Strawberries	6. Asparagus
7. Cherries	7. Sweet Peas
8. Kale	8. Kiwi
9. Lettuce	9. Cabbage
10. Grapes (Imported)	10. Eggplant
11. Carrots	11. Papaya
12. Pears	12. Watermelon
	13. Broccoli
	14. Tomato
	15. Sweet Potato

(Environmental Working Group)

Why Should You Care About Pesticides?
The growing consensus among scientists is that small doses of pesticides and other chemicals can cause lasting damage to human health, especially during fetal development and early childhood. Scientists now know enough about the long-term consequences of ingesting these powerful chemicals to advise that we minimize our consumption of pesticides.

What's the Difference?
EWG research has found that people who eat the twelve most contaminated fruits and vegetables consume an average of ten pesticides a day. Those who eat the fifteen least contaminated, conventionally-grown fruits and vegetables ingest fewer than two pesticides daily. The Guide helps consumers make informed choices to lower their dietary pesticide load.

Will Washing and Peeling Help?
Nearly all the studies used to create these lists assume that people rinse or peel fresh produce. Rinsing reduces but does not eliminate pesticides. Peeling helps, but valuable nutrients often go down the drain with the skin. The best approach: Eat a varied diet, rinse all produce, and buy organic when possible.

For further information, visit
The Environmental Working Group
www.foodnews.org
www.ewg.org

Chapter 8

The Fridge and Pantry

Every kitchen needs to be stocked with staple items so that meals can be prepared quickly and efficiently. If you enjoy preparing food and are already a cooking pro, you know that having the items readily available is very important. If you are just getting to know your kitchen better, this is where you must start — gathering the essentials.

Here is a list of recommended items to help get you started:

THE PANTRY		
Extra Virgin Olive Oil	Buckwheat	Curry Powder
Coconut Oil	Millet	Coconut Flour
Coconut Milk	Chicken Broth	Grass Fed Whey Protein
Coconut Flakes	Beans (black beans, chickpeas, kidney beans, etc dry or canned)	Whole Oatmeal
Tamari or Liquid Aminos	Canned tomatoes (crushed, diced)	Dried Fruits
Brown Rice	Gomasio (sesame seeds & seaweed)	Pure (Baker's) chocolate
Quinoa	All-purpose natural seasoning	Herbs and Spices
Buckwheat	Cajun Spice	Sea Salt
Stevia and Xylitol		

THE COUNTER	
Ripening avocados	Ripening bananas
Ripening fresh fruit	Ripening tomatoes
Growing sprouts	

THE FRIDGE		
Apple Cider Vinegar	Raw Nuts	Free-range Eggs
Almond Milk (unsweetened)	Hemp Milk	Hemp Seeds
Flax Seeds and Ground Flax Meal	Fruit Sweetened Ketchup	Olives (green, black, kalamata)
Flax Seed Oil	Butter	Yogurt
Kefir	Salsa	Hemp Seed Oil
Grape Seed Oil Vegenaise® (acceptable mayonnaise substitute)		

THE FREEZER	
Frozen Berries	Frozen Bananas and other fruits
Ginger	Whole Grain/Sprouted Breads, Bagels, English Muffins, etc.

MEATS/FISH	
Naturally raised chicken and turkey	Grass-fed beef
Grass-fed bison	Wild fish
Wild game	Turkey Bacon
Deli Meats	

Chapter 9

In the Kitchen

Many people love to cook but may unknowingly be preparing meals that are harmful by using unhealthy ingredients and incorrect cooking procedures. You don't have to look far to find 24-hour food channels in which 23 hours are typically dedicated to the preparation of pastas, breads, and white foods — not to mention bad fats and desserts. Even eating at home has become an exercise in convenience and speed when television shows boast how quickly each meal can be made. We need to reprogram our thinking and get back to the basics.

For those of you new to the kitchen, you may want to brush up on the function and how-to's of your stovetop and oven. The following simple tips will get you up and running quickly. For those of you already comfortable in the kitchen, you will find out how simple it is to prepare meals according to the Three Core Principles of the Maximized Living Nutrition Plans.

Kitchen Equipment

Your kitchen doesn't have to be elaborate — nor do you have to invest a lot of money in order to prepare a Maximized Meal.

Here is a list of affordable, everyday items you would need in any kitchen, regardless of the food you are making

Knives	Pepper grinder
Kitchen shears / scissors	Spatulas and tongs
Vegetable peeler	Measuring cups and spoons
Salad spinner	Mixing bowls
Citrus juicer or reamer	Colander/strainer
Garlic press	Cutting boards

In order to make the most of your kitchen encounters with minimal effort, additional investments may be necessary. However, each of the following small appliances is available in varying sizes and quality. There are $11 travel blenders all the way to the top-of-the-line

Vita-Mix®. Your choices will depend on your need and use of the following:

Food Processor – efficient way to chop and puree vegetables to create quick salads, spreads, dips, soups, and snacks.

Blender – good for smoothies and soups. Some high-end blenders, such as the Vita-Mix, double as a food processor.

Crock Pot – cooks food slowly. Place all your ingredients in the crock pot in the morning and come home to a hot meal. You can make meals large enough to have plenty of left-overs. Crock pots are terrific for slow-cooking roasts and whole chickens.

Indoor Grill – when it's not barbeque season, use a cast-iron grill for the safest and least toxic form of indoor grilling.

Steamer – the healthiest way to cook your vegetables. Gently steam them in either an electric steamer or a steamer basket over a pan.

Food Dehydrator – if set on 150ºF or less, the food retains its raw, live qualities.

Cookware (including grill pans and a heavy bottomed soup pot) - the safest and least toxic forms of cookware are cast iron and enameled cast iron, followed by stainless steel, Thermolon™ and glass. Newer brands of non-stick ceramic cookware are not only non-toxic but easy to use in place of traditional non-stick cookware. (Teflon® is facing class-action lawsuits and possible extinction within the next decade due to toxicity hazards.)

The following items, which are not considered essentials, may come in handy, depending on how creative you get

Vegetable spiral slicer – transform zucchini into pasta instantly. Without the skins, you won't be able to tell the difference. Cook in any sauce and you've effectively replaced traditional carbohydrates with healthy vegetables. The spiral slicer is also ideal for creative salad toppings, such as carrots and onions.

Citrus juicer or reamer

One-quart mason jars and lids for storing and soaking ingredients

Fine mesh strainer

Sprout bag – makes growing sprouts a cinch.

Microplane® - great for whole nutmeg, ginger, and citrus peels, etc

Roaster pan

Mortar/pestle – blending spices is one of the best ways to ensure a constant variety of flavors in the kitchen.

Juicer – if you find yourself doing more juicing than your blender can handle, an actual vegetable-and-fruit juicer is an incredible tool to create delicious drinks to nourish the whole family.

Kitchen Tips

- Clean out and reorganize your pantry and refrigerator. Now that you know which foods belong in your body, start with a clean slate and remove anything that is hazardous to your health.

- Set up a flow for your kitchen so that your glasses are near the dishwasher, colanders are by the sink, and pots and pans are by the stove.

- Keep you favorite recipes organized and easily accessible in the kitchen.

- Eliminate what you don't need. Try the "box rule." Put all your kitchen gadgets and utensils in a large, plastic bin or cardboard box. Pull items from the box as you need them. At the end of thirty days, discard what is left in the box. Or at least keep those items somewhere else in the house, because you obviously don't use them frequently nor need them within arm's reach.

- Leave your favorite and most-used gadgets on the counter. If you make smoothies every day, leave the blender on the countertop. If you are using your food processor often, find a convenient and accessible place for it so you aren't wasting time and energy. You'll be more encouraged to use your kitchen tools if it doesn't seem like work.

- Clean up as you go. It is much easier to put things away and load the dishwasher while your meal is simmering, than to have to clean up everything after a meal.

- Keep it fun. Turn on the music. Involve the entire family!

Meal Preparation and Time-Saving Tips

- Chop, wash, and bag your vegetables at the beginning of the week. This keeps bell peppers, onions, celery, broccoli, cucumbers, and lettuce within reach for a quick salad or snack. (Keep foods like tomatoes and strawberries whole and un-bagged until you need them, because they don't do as well stored.)

- Cook once for multiple meals. Prepare large enough meals on Saturday and Sunday so you will have easy leftovers for the week ahead.

MAXIMIZED LIVING COOKING POINTERS

Vegetables and Fruits:
- Incorporate as many raw vegetables as possible into your diet.

- Do not overcook when steaming vegetables. Aim for the vegetables to retain their vibrant colors and remain slightly crisp.

- Drizzle olive oil, avocado oil or walnut oil over the vegetables right after they are steamed for extra nutrition and flavor. Sea salt, pepper, garlic, butter, and other spices will add additional taste and variety.

- Try "steam frying" your vegetables for safe "browning." Add a small amount of oil to a pan and cook for 60 seconds. Add some water to the pan. Some people also like to add tamari or lemon juice. Cover with a lid and cook until vegetables are brown.

- Roast Brussels sprouts, leeks, onions, celery, eggplant, fennel, radicchio, squash, and zucchini in the oven. These are the best vegetables for roasting.

- Grill vegetables on an indoor grill. Coat the vegetables with olive oil and herbs for additional flavor. This method is wonderful for fajitas.

- Remember when purchasing vegetables: 1) fresh is best, 2) frozen is next best, and 3) canned is the last resort

Berries

- Enjoy fresh, summer berries all year long by freezing them. They are a great addition to smoothies, breakfasts, and healthy desserts; and they will last twelve to eighteen months after freezing.

- Use freezer-grade containers or bags for the best results. If you prefer to use regular plastic containers or bags, line them with parchment or waxed paper.

- Leave a 1-inch space at the top when packing food into containers. When packing the berries into bags, leave 2-4 inches at the top and then squeeze out the air to allow for expansion during freezing. Label, date, and freeze the berries.

- Thaw frozen berries in the refrigerator. For immediate use, thaw the container in cold water.

Freezing Bananas

- Freeze bananas whole. They keep well in the freezer and are great in workout smoothies.

- Blend frozen bananas with vanilla and coconut milk for a healthy ice cream-like treat.

- Peel the bananas before freezing, and then place them in a freezer bag lined with parchment paper. Slice before blending.

Poultry:

- Roasting and poaching are the best methods for cooking poultry.

  - **Roasting directions.** Season the whole chicken and put it in the oven at 350°F. Cook until a meat thermometer shows the internal temperature of the chicken is 170°F-180°F. A general rule of thumb is twenty minutes per pound of meat, with ten to twenty minutes of additional cooking time at 350°F.

  - Approximate Roasting Times for Chicken

2 ½ lbs -3 lbs : 1 to 1 ¾ hrs	4 ½ lbs – 5 lbs: 1 ½ to 2 hrs
3 ½ lbs – 4 lbs : 1 ½ to 3/4 hrs	5 – 6 lbs : 1 ¾ – 2 ½ hrs

  - Approximate Roasting Times for Turkey

Unstuffed	Stuffed
8-12 lbs : 2 ¾ – 3 hrs	3 – 3 ½ hrs
12-14 lbs :3 – 3 ¾ hrs	3 ½ – 4 hrs

Unstuffed	Stuffed
14 - 18 lbs : 3 ¾ - 4 ¼ hrs	4 - 4 ¼ hrs
18 - 20 lbs: 4 ¼ - 4 ½ hrs	4 ¼ - 4 ¾ hrs
20 - 24 lbs: 4 ⅕ hrs	4 ¾ - 5 ¼ hrs

- **Poaching directions.** Place the chicken into boiling water, with or without chicken or vegetable stock, and cook until it is no longer pink in the middle. This will take about fifteen to twenty minutes for chicken pieces; forty-five to sixty minutes for a whole chicken. You can add seasoning to the boiling water for added flavor. Poaching is perfect when you want chicken for tacos or salads.

• Sauté or stir fry chicken with coconut oil, butter, olive oil, or grape seed oil. Use a non-toxic, non-stick (non-Teflon®), or stainless steel pan.

Red Meats:

• Grass-fed red meats are lean causing them to cook quicker than grain-fed beef, which has a lot of fatty insulation. Therefore, to keep grass-fed beef tender, you must cook it slowly.

• The best method of cooking beef is slow roasting in the oven or crock pot. Be sure to first sear the beef to lock in the juices before placing it in a preheated oven.

• When grilling or broiling, first sear the beef, then lower the heat, (or keep the meat further away from the heat source), and turn it frequently. Do not overcook.

• You can coat the outsides of the meat with healthy oils to enhance flavor and to prevent sticking.

• Marinating beef before cooking helps to tenderize the meat.

• Grass-fed beef typically needs about 30 percent less cooking time than conventional meat. It is ideal to eat grass-fed beef medium rare. Do not cook well done.

Rare	130 – 140°F
Medium rare	140 – 145°F
Medium	145 - 155°F
Medium Well	155 - 160°F
Well Done	160 - 170°F

Cooking With Oils

HIGH HEAT: Use only coconut oil, olive oil, grape seed oil, or rice bran oil for frying. The best choice is coconut oil because of its superior flavor when frying foods such as chicken, not to mention its healthy benefits. Olive oil, while just as healthy, tends to make food soggy rather than crispy. A word of caution regarding olive oil: It will turn rancid when heated above 120°F. If it smokes, it has already turned rancid.

MEDIUM HEAT: To sauté foods, use sesame oil, rice bran oil, olive oil, grape seed oil, coconut oil, butter, or clarified butter (ghee). Note: Butter has turned rancid once it browns.

BAKING: Butter, coconut oil, sunflower oil, safflower oil, or olive oil can be used in baking if the temperature is less than 325°F. In a hotter oven, use only butter, olive oil, or coconut oil. When coating a pan or cookie sheet, use only coconut oil or grape seed oil.

Cooking with Flax Oil and Flax Seed Meal

Cold-pressed oils, such as flaxseed oil and hemp seed oil, should never be heated or used for frying. But they can be added to foods once they are cooked. These healthy oils can be added to stews, soups, sauces, salad dressings, casseroles, and nut butter to add nutritional value and flavor. They should be refrigerated at all times.

Although flaxseed oil, once extracted, should never be heated on its own, numerous studies have shown flax seeds and ground flax meal (milled flax seeds) is stable when cooked. Even when heated at 350°F for one hour, no changes occur to the peroxide values or fatty acid composition. (Ratnayake, et al, *Journal of Nutritional Biochemistry 3.)* This makes ground flax meal an excellent and acceptable flour substitute in our Advanced Plan recipes.

Chapter 10

Meals on the Go

The Lunchbox

You're at work, and it's lunchtime. You only have thirty minutes before your next meeting, and you didn't bring lunch with you. Now you know why donut shops do such a big business and why so many co-workers are gaining weight.

You've been invited to a staff lunch. And although there is an abundance of staff, there is a deficiency of anything you would consider a real lunch.

You've skipped meals all day, and you have a half-hour before you need to pick up your children from school. You are sitting in your van in rush-hour traffic, and every sign you see has the image of a burger on it.

You're out of town for the day. Nothing packed. The closest thing in sight that resembles a grocery store or restaurant is the nacho cheese pump at the gas station

Nothing is worse than being in a spot where you are hungry and not having a plan. Chances are that you will stop at the nearest drive-through or head to the vending machines. **Neither of these options is a plan. They are reactions to not having a plan.**

In today's world, having a plan may be just as important as the plan itself. **When you fail to plan, you plan to fail.**

Commit to the action steps in this book, and you will change your life and your family's future for the better, forever.

Consider what an incredible gift that would be to you and those you love. But that gift will require planning and preparation, especially when you leave the safety of your own home, or your Maximized Living Health Center, and step into a world that is in desperate need of help.

The Time Factor

For a working mother of three, attending three sporting practices per week, the temptation of microwave meals and drive-through restaurants can be overpowering. But at what cost? Excuses are dangerous and are no match for sickness and disease. And while no one is suggesting that the fast-paced meals of the 21st-century are good for you, there is a recurring excuse that they save time and money. Are you sure?

Imagine this same mom, knowing that she was going to be on-the-go and short on time, packed a cooler filled with fruit, sliced chicken, pre-made salads, and some water with lemon slices. Toting it to a picnic table at the ball field would allow her to feed everyone a healthy lunch or dinner, and it's even faster than going to the drive-through restaurant. Is this type of planning and preparation always easy? NO. It takes attention and commitment, but it can be done. For your health and the health of your family, it must be done.

You either eat healthy or you don't. The outcome will be good or bad. There are direct consequences for either decision. But ultimately, the decision is yours to make.

Cook for Multiple Meals – and Take Leftovers

If it takes you twenty minutes to prepare a typical meal, why not prepare several meals at the same time on Saturday or Sunday afternoon to last you for the week?

For example: Instead of cooking two filets of salmon, cook six. Use the leftovers for a salmon salad you can take to work, bring on the road, or leave in the refrigerator for those moments when you're hungry. Multiple-meal preparation may cause you to spend an extra hour chopping, cooking, and bagging up food for the week; but that hour will save you several others.

When you get home late after a busy day, you'll be glad you invested the time to prepare food that can be put on your plate in five minutes. Add steamed vegetables to cold leftovers or a pre-made salad, and it will taste like a fresh hot meal in a fraction of the time.

Simple Supplements

Ideally, we would love to have all meals beautifully prepared and served on a china plate. However, whether you travel, have multiple jobs, or spend long days outside the home, chances are not every one of your meal times will turn out this way.

Unfortunately, the overwhelming majority of meal replacements available in grocery stores, vending machines, and gas stations are loaded with preservatives, sugar, and bad fats — including bars that claim to be healthy.

It's not that difficult to prepare your own meal replacements, using the simple supplements referenced in Chapter 12. For example, in a glass jar, pack some healthy whey or hemp protein mixed with high-quality greens powder. When you are hungry, simply add clean water and mix yourself a shake on the spot. While traveling, take a container of a recommended healthy meal replacement, and some other pure foods listed below, then you'll never be caught unprepared or unnourished.

Fiber and Good Fats Keep You Full!

Some of the best snacks to keep in your lunchbox include:

Raw nuts and seeds. If you wish, season them with sea salt or pepper for some variety.	Olives, Coconut, Avocados - these fats are vital at the cellular level and will keep you full for hours.

Sliced, high-fiber veggies such as broccoli and celery.	Raw Cheeses.
100 percent sprouted grain tortillas.	Full-fat Yogurt.
Homemade trail mix.	Homemade protein bars and muffins (See recipes beginning on page 105).
Whey or hemp protein powder to mix up a quick shake.	Quality greens powder for a refreshing and energizing drink.

A freezer pack is recommended to keep homemade snack bars, yogurts, cheeses, and vegetables cold.

Lunches for the Children — and for You!

As the health of the Western world plummets, increasing numbers of children are developing allergies to nuts and eggs, making lunchbox options much more restricted. These children will be entering the workforce in ten years, and soon you'll have difficulty packing what you want to bring to work. While Maximized Living is helping thousands of children overcome their allergies and hypersensitivities, please consider the following suggestions when packing lunches in order to keep from creating additional health problems for others:

Soups (most soups can be eaten cold).	Raw cheeses and yogurt.
Hummus (or other homemade dip) with sliced vegetables.	Shredded carrots with oil and vinegar.
100 percent sprouted grain crackers or grain-free (seed) crackers.	Spiral-sliced zucchini or squash with natural pesto sauce.
Salads – the options are endless, and the vegetables will fill you up. See meal ideas in Chapter 6.	Artichokes.
Beef jerky, turkey jerky, salmon salad.	Berries.
Sardines and anchovies.	

When you prepare nourishing, satisfying lunches, the number one consideration is excluding anti-nutrients, such as sugar and white flour (i.e. soda crackers), which deplete your nutrient sources, spike your insulin, and actually make you hungrier.

Chapter 11

The Restaurant

Eating Out

North Americans are notorious for eating out. We go out for the food, the entertainment, the fun, and the convenience. But to the detriment of far too many, this has become a life-style habit difficult to overcome. When "too busy" is the family motto, eating out becomes the norm; and the restaurant or food court takes the place of the dining room table.

The Real Cost

We're not saying "never eat out." We do encourage you, however, to add up the cost of eating out — to your pocketbook and to your health. It is estimated that 42 percent of Americans' food budgets and 30 percent of Canadians' are spent in restaurants. Dollars spent to eat out in the United Kingdom just surpassed the amount spent for meals in the home. (National Statistics, London, England.)

Statistics show the average household now makes 500-700 trips annually to restaurants. Let's do the math: Take a family that visits a restaurant for a $4 snack, five days a week; and add a $35 family meal twice a week. That household is spending $4,680 per year at restaurants.

The traditional argument is that eating out costs less than buying healthy food to prepare at home. Are you sure?

Consider These Ways to Save on Your Grocery Bill:
- Go natural and organic, especially when buying animal products and those items with the highest pesticide load. (See Chapter 8, page 81.) But your entire pantry does not need to be organic.

- Eliminate foods that you now know are detrimental to your health. Most people will see see their grocery bill expenses drop by taking this step.

- Order food directly from local farmers, local co-ops, or other healthy sources, and bypass the "middle man."

Portion Sizes
It is also important to consider portion sizes -- a major concern when eating out. Most

restaurant portions are two to three times greater than a normal portion should be. Since most people don't like to waste money, they will eat what is put on their plate, no matter what size it is. We have been conditioned to think that super-sized meals have more value. "The bigger, the better" has had devastating consequences. The ultimate price you will pay with your health deserves serious consideration.

For example, a reasonable portion of pasta should be about 1 cup or 1½ cups. When we make or order pasta, we typically eat from a Frisbee®-sized plate with a large mound of pasta and sauce. On top of that we add salad, bread, and possibly even an appetizer and dessert. This is harsh punishment for our bodies. Contrast that to Europe, where portion sizes are typically one-third the size served in North America.

What we really require are smaller and more nourishing meals that provide adequate amount of fats, proteins, and nutrients that will keep you full and feeling satisfied for several hours. If you are doing it right, you will never feel like you are starving.

Here are some helpful guidelines to follow when it comes to portion sizes:

- Protein: 1 serving = the size of one fist
- Green vegetables or salad greens: 1 serving = the size of two fists
- Starchy carbohydrates: 1 serving = the size of your fist. (Should be eaten in the daytime and in moderation on the Core Plan only.)

While these amounts may seem modest, realize your stomach is only about the size of two fists loosely held together. It is important to listen to your body, and this is where most people falter. Eating slowly allows your brain time to trigger its "I'm full" response. There is about a twenty-minute delay in this feeling, which makes it easy to overindulge. If your plate is not yet empty, take some home for tomorrow's lunch or dinner.

Fast Food or the Family Restaurant?
The only people in the food industry who suggest that fast food has any benefit are those in the fast-food industry — and their marketing departments. There hasn't been a single study yet suggesting otherwise. However, don't assume that sit-down, full-service restaurants are always a healthier option, because the food served at those restaurants is mostly dressed up fast food. Instead of standing in line, you sit at a table. It comes on a plate instead of in a bag. But when you check the ingredient list and the way the food is prepared, Your Neighborhood Grill, and the place where you get your baby backs, are no better than a typical fast-food restaurant.

The Biggest Problem: What's in the Food?
Whether on a tight or unlimited budget, the biggest concern should be what goes into those delectable-looking dishes displayed on the menu. Restaurants typically focus on taste - not health - because they want you to come back. Most of our taste buds have been under attack for decades. And yes, bad fats and sugar taste good.

Many restaurants are moving away from using trans fats, some mandated by law. Others are now starting to put "heart smart" items on their menu, and even partner with gyms to list "cardio-friendly" meals. These trends are part of the solution, but not the entire answer, because their definitions of healthy are primarily based on calorie counts and portion size.

By these standards, you might as well just have a low-calorie chocolate bar for dinner. But no one would suggest that is healthy.

Until restaurants are required to deliver the Maximized Living seal of approval on menu items, here are some hints to help you when you go out to eat:

War Plan

- Plan what you are going to eat before you get there. Many restaurants have their menus online so it is easy to check in advance.

- Attribute special requests to allergies rather than being picky. You may not have been diagnosed specifically with the condition. But at the cellular level, we are all allergic to sugar and bad fats. Many of us are pre-diabetic from years of the Standard North American Diet. In our experience, restaurants are more accommodating to customers with special health concerns and conditions.

- Scan the menu. If asparagus appears somewhere on the menu, but is not included with the item you are ordering, ask to substitute it for something else. It's worth the extra charge, if there is one.

- Ask if they use margarine or butter. Many large chains think it's the same thing. The same misunderstanding applies to canola oil versus olive oil. With rising food costs, restaurants often use the cheapest options, which are not healthy fats, such as butter and olive oil.

- Have children order off the adult menu, and then have them share. Typically, there is nothing healthy on a children's menu.

What to Avoid
- Skip the bread and butter before your meal. In fact, ask them not to even bring it to the table.

- Avoid soups, especially cream-based soups. Soups are notorious for hiding harmful ingredients, such as MSG (monosodium glutamate), excess table salt, and hydrogenated oils. Most soups come in large bags, pre-made at a manufacturing plant, loaded with additives and preservatives, and then shipped for hundreds of miles. They are not exactly mom's homemade soup.

- Skip the appetizers. Instead, start with a salad, but be careful. Restaurant salad dressings are loaded with nutrition-killers, such as bad oils, sugars, salt, and additives. They can cause a salad to have more bad fats and bad calories than a hamburger and French fries. Request olive oil and vinegar or olive oil and lemon slices for your dressing. Most restaurants will accommodate this. You can even bring small packs of your own dressing to restaurants. You're only saving them money so they typically won't mind.

- Skip dessert. When following the Maximized Living Nutrition Plans, and including plenty of good fats, you won't likely be hungry.

What to Order
- Make your own salad creation. If you see any ingredients on the menu that would make a good salad, ask them to make you one. For instance, combine grilled onions and peppers with broccoli, artichokes, or black beans.

- Substitute a second vegetable for starchy carbohydrates, such as potatoes or rice.

- Ask for foods to be baked, grilled, or broiled — not fried.

- Ask for a plate of raw vegetables. Many restaurants have vegetables chopped and ready to go into other dishes. The addition of high-fiber, raw vegetables to any meal will help you fill up, making it easier to skip the dessert.

- Ask for all sauces on the side. Better yet, don't include them with your meal, because they usually contain harmful ingredients. If you do choose to eat sauces, simply drizzle a few drops; don't slather it on like the restaurants do.

- Squeeze lemon slices over your meal for extra flavor.

- Keep sea salt in your jacket or purse as an alternative to table salt.

- Lamb is often grass-fed, specifically if it is from New Zealand, so it is a great meat option when eating out.

- Turkey can be less toxic than commercial chicken, because it is not mass-produced as often. However, this is only a guideline.

- If you are ordering fish, make sure it was caught in the wild and preferably not from the Atlantic Ocean due to toxicity issues. If the server or manager does not know the source, order something else. Most restaurants serve farm-raised fish.

- Always drink water, preferably bottled, with your meal. This will save you a lot of money. Most restaurants charge $1-$3 for sodas, lemonades, and specialty drinks, which are all primarily liquid sugar.

Don't feel like you have to finish everything. Restaurants give you way too much food. Most meals are 2-3 times bigger than a normal serving size. Save half for lunch the next day or split your dish with someone else. Get in the habit of taking some of the food home.

Look for organic restaurants that accommodate the Maximized Living Nutrition Plans. Search online for options in your area. Your Maximized Living office may also have some recommendations.

You also can check the nutrition facts of your favorite dishes online. This is sometimes provided by the restaurant or by independent research. Go to thedailyplate.com to check entrees at specific restaurants.

These are just some ideas to get you started. Our hope is that you will reduce the amount of time spent eating out. And when you do go out, we hope you will make MAXIMIZED decisions. If more people demand healthier foods, the restaurants will respond. If they notice that their hormone- and antibiotic-filled fried chicken tenders with hydrogenated oil soaked French fries are not popular choices, they will take them off the menu.

We look forward to the day when we can all go to restaurants that understand and implement the Five Essentials of Maximized Living. It may be another few decades before we are there. Until then, let's keep sharing the vision with others, for our benefit and theirs.

Eating at Home – The Benefits

Choosing to eat home-cooked meals provides the following benefits:
- You get to decide the ingredients.
- You can take pride in nourishing yourself and your family.
- You can spend quality time preparing the meal and eating with your family without the distractions of a busy, noisy restaurant.
- It will save you time and money.
- You can use a home-cooked meal to entertain friends, while introducing them to Maximized Living principles. This may save their lives!
- It will save your life, too.

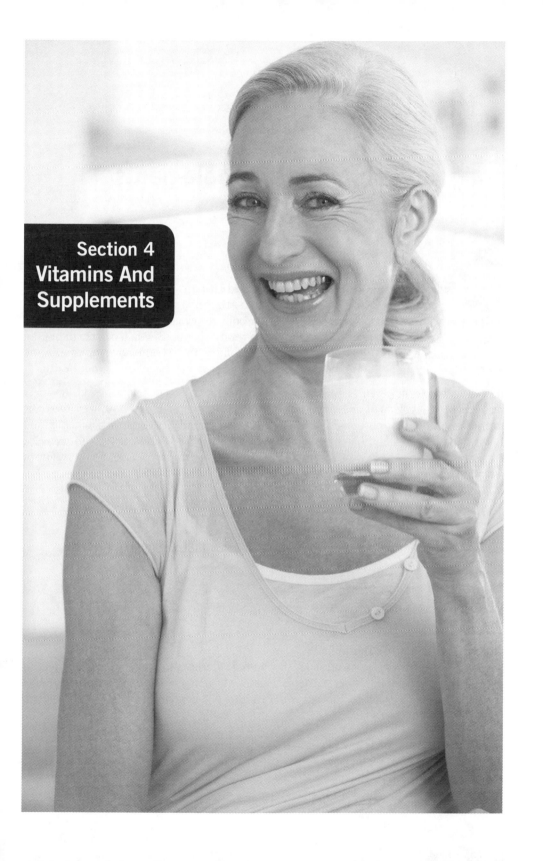

**Section 4
Vitamins And
Supplements**

Chapter 12

Vitamins and Supplements

By now you're beginning to realize that Maximized Living is not just another promotion, program, or gimmick — it's a revolutionary way to attain and sustain health and healing. If it were not for the depletion of nutrients from our soils, the evolution of genetically-modified foods, and the introduction of chemical toxins in foods, your body would be able to get the vital nutrients it needs from foods alone. Unfortunately, that is no longer the case in the 21st century. So, proper supplements are a vital component of establishing your health.

It's not as simple, however, as asking the clerk at the grocery store or purchasing the latest recommended supplement and vitamin you read about in a magazine. You need the right nutrients, in the right portions, and from the right sources. These vitamins, minerals, and herbs can boost immunity and give you the nutrients necessary for repair and recovery. They also help your body deal with issues of toxicity, weakness, damage, and breakdown from unknown, long-term nutritional deficiencies and poor bodily function.

The Do's and Don'ts for Vitamins and Supplements

Do take vitamins and supplements to provide the nutrition that is no longer present in our food.

(New England Journal of Medicine)

We would love to get all of our nutrition from foods, but that simply isn't possible in today's world. Some of the reasons include:

Nutrients in Foods Are Declining
Evidence is everywhere telling us about the dramatic declines in the nutritional content of our fruits and vegetables. Fewer nutrients mean we have to eat more fruits and vegetables to derive the same benefits. This is a worldwide phenomenon. (Lerner, et al, *Maximized Living Makeover.)*

The Toxins in Some of Today's Foods Are Increasing
The omega-3 fatty acids found in fish are absolutely essential for overall health. But the pollution of lakes, rivers, and oceans means it's actually dangerous to consume the amount of fish necessary to get the fish oil we require. This leads us to fish oil capsules derived from cold-water fish that have been filtered for purity. It's simply the only safe way.

The Foods Most Easily Available to Us Are Designed with One Thing in Mind – Sell

It's not exactly a news flash to observe that the Standard North American Diet is designed more to optimize corporate profits and market share than to provide healthy, nutritious food. (Lerner, et al, *Maximized Living Makeover.*)

Organic Food – Better, but Not Always Accessible and Usually More Expensive

You should try to eat organic as much as possible, starting at the top of the food chain as described in the Core Plan. However, in today's world of fast-food eating and tight budgets, you'll still need vitamins and supplements to close the nutritional gap.

Don't Take Vitamins and Supplements to Treat Diseases

As North Americans, we are raised from the earliest age to be pill-poppers. Naturally, we assume that if we want to be healthier, we need to swallow a pill. But popular opinion is turning strongly toward a natural approach. The world is beginning to realize that taking prescription medication for our health problems is not only minimally effective but also is poisoning our bodies. Many people have started turning to nutrition and supplements as a better choice than drugs. What they don't realize is they are still using nutrition as medicine to cure a symptom.

Many lead the same lifestyle, and do not change their fundamental approach on how they deal with their health. When they get headaches, they'll pop vitamin B-12 tablets instead of aspirins and think they are doing their bodies a favor. Or they say they do not want to take medication for their indigestion but will take herbs instead. The truth is whether you take medication or a supplement to treat a symptom, you have the same result.

Just because you can buy a supplement without a prescription at the grocery store doesn't mean that it's safe for you. For instance, we've all heard of beta-carotene. It's an antioxidant that is good for fighting cancer. But it turns out that if you put beta-carotene in most pill forms, it's actually toxic and causes cancer.

Chasing good health based on symptoms is confusing, contradictory, even dangerous, and will most likely get you nowhere. If you want a more effective way of using the natural approach, do not take a nutritional supplement for the purpose of treating a symptom or condition. The most effective way of avoiding aches, pains, sickness, and disease in the first place is to follow the Maximized Living lifestyle that provides the body the nutrition it needs through real foods, vitamins, and supplements.

Don't Take Vitamins and Supplements in Place of Food

Researchers from the Harvard School of Public Health noted that "a vitamin supplement cannot begin to compensate for the massive risks associated with smoking, obesity, or inactivity." (Willett and Stampfer, *The New England Journal of Medicine*, 2002.) Supplements should be just that: supplements to the foods you eat each day — not a replacement for them.

Vitamins, Supplements and Your Body — What Has to Happen

We have to ingest them. As long as they're in a bottle, they're not helping anyone.

We have to absorb them. Just because there is the same amount of a vitamin in a cheap multivitamin as in a premium, pharmaceutical-grade multivitamin doesn't necessarily mean they are absorbed by the body equally as well.

We have to utilize them. One of the most important concepts to understand is that by following The 5 Essentials of Maximized Living, you will empower your body's ability to remove anything that interferes with your innate healing system. Maximized Living doctors make sure your nerve supply, oxygen, lean muscle mass, detoxification, and peace of mind are in harmony. That way your body will function at a peak level. Your doctor also can help you choose the right supplements.

Special Focus: Vitamin D

Even if you follow the strictest of diets, chances are you are deficient in Vitamin D. The major contributor to the activation of this vital force in your immune system is not any one food, but your daily exposure to the sun's rays.

Vitamin D is a major component for maintaining bone density and strength and helps to absorb much needed calcium from the intestines. A lack of Vitamin D causes calcium-depleted bones, which increases the risk of fractures due to weak bones. Millions of North Americans lack a sufficient amount of Vitamin D in their blood to protect their bones. The current recommended daily intake for Vitamin D runs from 200-600 IU's per day, depending on your age. However, in light of recent research, and with most people testing "severely deficient" in blood testing today, this level of supplementation seems to be inadequate.

Vitamin D concentration in the body is correlated with immune function (i.e. fighting off the flu and preventing cancer), and contributes in multiple ways to the optimal function of the human body as virtually every cell has a receptor for Vitamin D. This includes the cells of the pancreas where vitamin D has its impact on blood sugar.

Vitamin D2 vs. Vitamin D3

If you are like most North Americans, the form of Vitamin D you are most likely lacking, and with which you need to supplement, is Vitamin D3 (cholecalciferol) – not Vitamin D2 (ergocalciferol). Vitamin D3 is not a vitamin in the traditional sense, but actually a pro-hormone that is produced in the skin from cholesterol in response to absorbing UVB rays. When this pro-hormone is converted via the liver, it is then transported to the kidneys and carried to the cell's nucleus, the heart of every cell, where it influences its physiology to take the healthy pathways by dictating genetic expression.

Most of us are lacking several thousand IU's of Vitamin D3 per day because we spend our days indoors – and even in the summer, we move from an air-conditioned house, to an air-conditioned car, to an air-conditioned office building, to an air-conditioned bedroom for the night ... Then we repeat the cycle the next day.

Blood Serum Levels of 25 Hydroxy Vitamin D

The level of Vitamin D circulating in our system is directly proportionate to the amount of skin exposed to sunlight. According to leading experts in medicine today, to have acceptable levels of 60-80 ng/mL we need 10-15 minutes of mid-day sun with 40% body exposure, and for most of us this is not possible.

Vitamin D Supplementation

Traditionally, people have been taught to supplement with 1000-2000 IU's of Vitamin D per day, to maintain levels above 20 ng/mL in order to prevent Rickets. Research compiled by Garland and Baggerly for GrassrootsHealth shows that levels should be at least 60 ng/mL to prevent diseases related to Vitamin D deficiency such as cancer, multiple sclerosis, and osteoporosis. Vitamin D testing often reveals that most people more accurately need to supplement with 5,000 for maintenance, or 10,000 IU per day until health levels are reached and verified by follow-up testing.

While it would be most ideal to get all the nutrients you need from food, the best source of D3 is the sun. In absence of regular sunlight, or in cases where body levels test lower than 60 ng/mL, be sure to supplement with a healthy form of Vitamin D3 on a daily basis. Other sources of D3 include salmon and mushrooms, but these do not provide nearly as much D3 as direct sunshine.

Three Keys to Safe and Effective Use of Vitamins and Supplements

Don't Skimp on Vitamins and Supplements

All vitamins and supplements are not created equal. Using discount and drugstore supplements is like swallowing stones. In order for the discount store to meet their profit margin, the wholesale price of these vitamins and supplements has to be low. What you pay is what you'll get.

If you need to economize, don't start with supplements. That would be like saving money on your transportation costs by neglecting regular oil changes. It will save you money in the short run but cost you much, much more in the long run. Similarly, saving a few pennies on your vitamins and supplements can ultimately mean spending hundreds of thousands or even millions more when you have to pay the healthcare consequences of sickness and disease.

Here's what you need to look for in a supplement:

Is it pharmaceutical grade or food grade? The best vitamins and supplements are manu-factured to exact pharmaceutical-grade standards ensuring the highest quality.

Is it organic? Just as you want your food to be organic, you should also insist on organically-derived ingredients for your vitamins and supplements.

Is it complete? Does it have the necessary range of nutrients that your body needs?

Is it potent? Does it have the nutrient in the minimum or optimum amount?

Is it bioavailable? Can your body easily absorb and utilize the nutrient?

Is it toxic? Vitamin A, for instance, can be toxic when taken in high doses over a long period of time.

Is it recommended by Maximized Living Doctors? They will probably recommend the same vitamins and supplements they take. They know firsthand that when combined with a comprehensive course of treatment, these vitamins and supplements consistently deliver. Your Maximized Living Doctor probably won't object if you insist on continuing to take your own supplements. But if you don't achieve the same dramatic results that other patients are receiving, then be open to taking the vitamins and supplements your doctor recommends.

Don't Take the Minimum Required. Take the Maximum Needed.

The Recommended Daily Intake (RDI) statistics you find on the label of your supplement aren't as helpful as they might seem. The fact that some vitamins have 600 percent or 3000 percent of the RDI of a certain nutrient is an acknowledgement that the RDI isn't enough. There are many reasons for this, but the fact of the matter is that the RDI doesn't take into account your age, gender, level of stress, health index, toxicity, degree of subluxation, and body composition. By consulting with your Maximized Living Doctor, you can put together a plan of action that's right for you.

Where to Start

Just taking an assortment of supplements will rarely ensure you get the ones your body needs. Additionally, it can be harmful because you might take too much of some and too little of others. We advise a basic protocol of supplements to support the Three Core Principles of the Maximized Living Nutrition Plan and to combat the modern challenges of today's foods.

Protein

The problem: Quality protein is hard to obtain.

The solution: Organic grass-fed whey supplement. Protein provides the building blocks for hormones and neurotransmitters. It is essential that you get an optimal amount of clean, lean protein at each meal. Cool-processed, grass-fed whey is a fantastic source of protein. It is bioavailable, raises the master antioxidant glutathione, and helps to bind and pull heavy metals out of the body. Be careful. Hydrolyzed and heat-processed whey proteins, which make up the majority of whey protein supplements on the market, do not contain the same benefits. Because their amino acids have been denatured through heat processing, they become virtually useless and potentially harmful in the body.

Sugar

The problem: Sugar and grains are the world's most popular carbohydrates. We all need a substantial amount of healthy, low-glycemic carbohydrates in our diets, but they can be sparse.

The solution: Greens drinks, also available in powder or capsules. Ideally, you need to eat five or more servings of colorful, raw, organic vegetables every day. These high-quality greens will ensure that you are getting what you need. In the absence of high vegetable intake, quality greens drinks can provide a synergistic blend of vegetable nutrients with no allergenic grains.

Fat

The problem: Fat is North America's number one missing ingredient. You need good fats — and lots of them — in the healthy ratios your body uses for function.

The solution: Omega-3 supplements. If you're eating a standard commercial diet that consists of little grass-fed meat, omega-3 eggs, walnuts, avocado, or fish, then you need to supplement the missing omega-3s in your diet. However, beware of two problems associated with omega-3 supplementation: It's common to overdo omega-3 supplementation and end up creating the opposite problem, omega-3 dominance. The other risk with fish oil supplements is mercury contamination from toxic waters. The best omega-3 supplements will not only give your body the ideal ratio of omega-3 and omega-6 fatty acids, but also will come from a blend of plant and fish sources, having been molecularly-filtered for optimum purity.

Toxins

The problem: Additives, preservatives, and chemicals are popping up everywhere — even in the healthiest foods.

The solution: Daily detoxification at the cellular level. Beware of fad cleanses, which actually rob the body of nutrients and may do more harm than good. Instead, consume the proper combination of amino acids, essential fats, and herbs daily to promote detoxification at the cellular level and to elevate glutathione, the body's own antioxidant and detoxifier. A complete detoxification system will do two things: 1) elevate your body's level of glutathione to escort toxins out of the cells, and 2) include a secondary component to permanently bind the fat-soluble toxins and remove them from the body. This will prevent so-called re-toxification, which is the most frequent and harmful complication of typical detoxification products found on the market today.

Nutrients

The problem: The erosion of soils has caused a depletion of nutrients in today's foods.

The solution: A multivitamin and/or multimineral supplement. Think of a high-quality, multivitamin/mineral and antioxidant formula as your proactive health insurance.

Get Expert Advice

Your Maximized Living Health Center is the ideal place to find the most updated information from practitioners who are helping hundreds of thousands of patients across North America establish health and experience Maximized Living. Maximized Living Doctors, along with their teams, are an invaluable resource. Let them assess your needs and lead you in the right direction. Without proper guidance, supplements can cause problems and are likely to be a huge waste of your time and money.

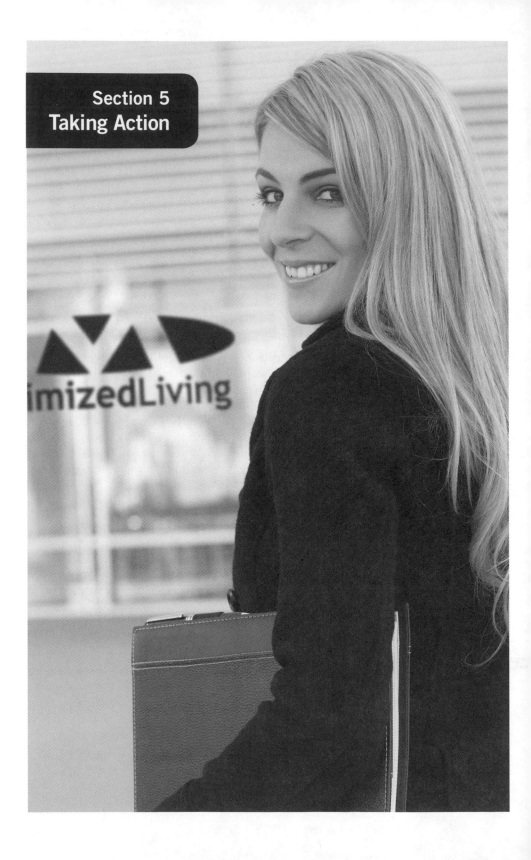

Section 5
Taking Action

Chapter 13

Taking Action

Following Through to a Long, Successful Life of Happy, Healthy Eating

A team of medical doctors and Ph.D's recently completed a study of U.S. adults who were 40-74 years old. The researchers compared the subjects' habits between 1988-1994 and 2001-2006. The results indicated that adherence to healthy habits dropped from 15 percent to 8 percent — from dismal to off-the-charts horrific. Of those studied, 92 percent were literally killing themselves. *(The American Journal of Medicine.)* These numbers are vital to consider before embarking on yet another attempt at a better lifestyle.

When it comes to following through, the biggest concern for nearly everyone is: "If I start eating well, can I keep eating well?"

The quick answer: "No, you can't do it."

Sounds negative, but sadly it's true for most of us. Even when people are told definitively, "Either make changes or die," they often still don't change.

The positive news is that there is a proven solution: Get help.

Studies done on the success of diet books revealed that, regardless of their claims, no diet — not even one — was successful long-term. This would explain that despite the sale of millions of diet resources, North Americans keep getting bigger and sicker. Some diet plans worked initially. But studies show that after one year the weight and overall health of participants on average was no better and often worse than when they started.

On the other hand, programs that involved a leader, accountability, and on-going education worked, and worked well. That's been our experience and our success. With proven, scientific nutritional information and programs, our patients get well and lose weight quickly. In addition, inspiring leadership, regular weigh-ins, continuing education through workshops and seminars, fitness challenges for every level, and the much-needed support from others making the same changes are all means to ensure success.

Dieting is never a game of being perfect. Setbacks are common. We expect them. They're called Vacation Meals, and we recommend them once or twice per week. It's not cheating. It's a part of eating, particularly when your goal is not just about dropping 15 pounds for the wedding or family reunion, but a fun, happy lifetime of joyful eating and long-term change.

Of course, there is much more to a Maximized life than just eating well. There are four other Maximized Living Essentials that you need to put into action if you expect to succeed. Our doctors will escort you through the process of making the necessary changes needed to reach your goals. The objective is to make your life easier and better, not harder.

The directory located at **maximizedliving.com** gives you a list of Maximized Living Doctors and clinics around the world. Look for a doctor certified in Essential #3: Maximized Quality Nutrition. These doctors have been trained by the authors of this book. Not only will you have access to them for support and advice, but you also will receive the most accurate and up-to-date information possible.

Your life will never be the same again. You now know that you have a choice about how you'll live the rest of your life. You can wake up every morning feeling refreshed and have the energy and clear mind to live joyfully. That is the life we want you to have. Accept our invitation and start living, really living, today.

www.MaximizedLiving.com

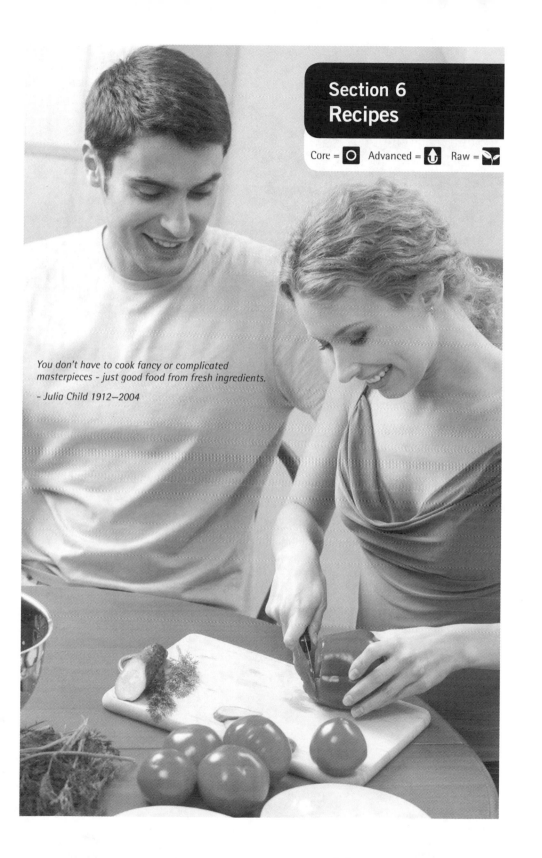

Section 6
Recipes

Core = O   Advanced = 🔱   Raw = 🌱

You don't have to cook fancy or complicated masterpieces - just good food from fresh ingredients.

- Julia Child 1912–2004

Breakfast

Spinach Omelette • Servings: 1

This is great for breakfast, lunch, or dinner and is very simple to make.

3-4 Eggs, Slightly Beaten
1 Cup Fresh Spinach
½ Cup Fresh Mushrooms
¼ Cup Onion, Chopped
⅛ Teaspoon Sea Salt
1 Tablespoon Coconut Oil

Tip: For an even fluffier omelette, add 1/3 cup water to the egg mixture before cooking. Mix thoroughly.

In a skillet, sauté the mushrooms, onions, and spinach leaves until tender, remove from the skillet. In a small bowl, stir together the remaining omelette ingredients except coconut oil. In the same skillet, heat coconut oil. Pour egg mixture into skillet. Cook over medium heat lifting slightly with spatula to allow uncooked portion to flow underneath until eggs are set (3-4 minutes). Place sautéed mushrooms, onion, and spinach on half of omelette. Gently fold over the other half and slide onto a plate.

Yogurt and Berries • Servings: 1

A great alternative for breakfast to replace cereal! It will keep you full and satisfied for hours!.

1 Cup Organic Full Fat Yogurt
½ Cup Fresh Blueberries or Raspberries
½ Teaspoon spoonable/powdered Stevia
1 Teaspoon Hemp Seed Oil (optional)
1-2 Tablespoons Whey Protein Powder (optional)

Stir all ingredients and serve immediately.

TIP: For added protein, add some whey protein powder.

TIP: Spoonable Stevia or 1:1 Stevia is equivalent to the same amount of sugar.

Eggs Florentine • Servings: 3-4

Eggs and spinach are a perfect flavor match.

2 Tablespoons Butter
½ Small Onion, Minced
1 Clove Minced Garlic
1 Lemon
1 Cups Spinach
6-8 Eggs

In a skillet, sauté onions and garlic in butter over medium heat. Once onions have started to soften, add spinach and allow it to wilt. Squeeze lemon over spinach. Scramble eggs and pour over mixture. Cook until eggs are done.

Free-range Eggs – Eggs are a versatile food which contain all 8 essential amino acids and are high in vitamins. Eggs are good for cancer prevention, the cardiovascular system, brain function, liver support, and cell membrane health. Eggs are high in the essential nutrient choline which helps prevent the accumulation of cholesterol in the liver.

Almond Power Bars • Servings: 8-10 Slices

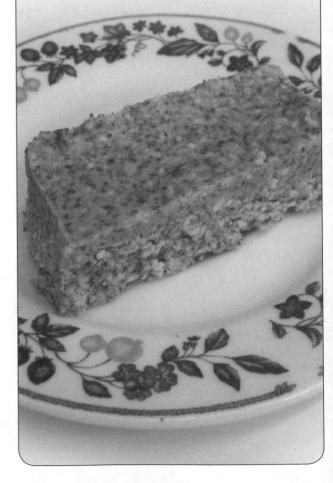

These no bake, high-protein, high-fiber bars are a cinch to make and easy to take along.

2 Cups Raw Almonds
$\frac{1}{2}$ Cup Flaxseed Meal
$\frac{1}{2}$ Cup Unsweetened Shredded Coconut
2 Scoops Flavored Whey Protein Powder
$\frac{1}{2}$ Cup Raw Almond Butter
$\frac{1}{2}$ Teaspoon Kosher Salt
$\frac{1}{2}$ Cup Coconut Oil
8 Drops Liquid Stevia or $\frac{3}{4}$ Teaspoon Stevia Powder, To Taste
1 tablespoon pure vanilla extract (No sugar – check the label)
8 squares unsweetened chocolate, melted and sweetened to taste with stevia and cinnamon (optional)

Place almonds, flax meal, shredded coconut, whey powder, almond butter and salt in a food processor. Pulse briefly, about 10 seconds. In a small sauce pan, melt coconut oil over very low heat.

Remove coconut oil from stove; stir stevia and vanilla into oil. Add coconut oil mixture to food processor and pulse until ingredients form a coarse paste. Press mixture into an 8 x 8 glass baking dish. (A parchment paper liner helps when you want to remove the bars from the dish.) Chill in refrigerator for 1 hour, until mixture hardens. In a double boiler, melt chocolate, stirring in stevia and cinnamon. Spread melted chocolate over bars; return to refrigerator for 30 minutes, until chocolate hardens. Remove from refrigerator, cut into bars, and serve.

These bars are pictured here naked for people who prefer to skip the chocolate coating.

TIP: Use other combinations of raw nuts and raw nut butters; such as macadamia.

Grain-free Pancakes • Servings: about 6 pancakes

You can still have the foods you enjoy, simply substitute healthy ingredients for unhealthy ones.

3 Eggs
3 Tablespoons Butter or Coconut Oil, Melted (plus extra butter or coconut oil for cooking the pancakes)
3 Tablespoons Coconut Milk or Whole Milk
$\frac{1}{2}$ Teaspoons Stevia or Xylitol
$\frac{1}{8}$ Teaspoon Sea Salt
2-4 Drops Pure Vanilla
3 Tablespoons Coconut Flour
$\frac{1}{2}$ Teaspoon Baking Powder

Using a wire whisk, mix together eggs, melted butter, milk, stevia, sea salt, and vanilla. Continuing to whisk, add the baking powder and coconut flour until thoroughly mixed. Heat 1 tablespoon of butter (or coconut oil) in a skillet on a medium flame. Spoon 2-3 tablespoons of batter onto skillet making pancakes about 3-4 inches in diameter. Sprinkle with bluberries if desired. Flip when pancakes start to form bubbles around the edges.

Optional: Blueberries, Strawberry Sauce (see recipe p. 159).

- -

Grainless Granola • Servings: 4

Great for those who miss their morning cereal.

$\frac{1}{4}$ Cup Whole Flaxseeds
$\frac{1}{4}$ Cup Raw Sunflower Seeds
$\frac{1}{4}$ Cup Raw Organic Almonds or Walnuts
$\frac{1}{4}$ Cup Raw Dehydrated Coconut Flakes, Unsweetened
$\frac{1}{2}$ Can Chilled Coconut Milk
$\frac{1}{4}$ Teaspoon Cinnamon

> TIP: This granola can be enjoyed cold or add coconut milk, let stand a few minutes, and warm slightly on stovetop for a hot cereal. Flax seeds will thicken mixture as it sits.

In a dry blender or food processor, pour flaxseeds, sunflower seeds, almonds, and coconut flakes through opening in top cover. Replace removable cap and continue processing until ingredients are reduced to a chunky, grain-like consistency, about 1 minute.

Stop motor, scrape down to loosen mixture in bottom of blender or work bowl, if necessary. Add cinnamon and process a few more bursts until blended.

Scoop out $\frac{1}{2}$ cup mixture per serving. Pour roughly equal amounts of coconut milk or other milk per serving over cereal and enjoy.

> _Berries_ – Berries are an incredible food. They lower inflammation and will not spike blood sugar. Like greens, they are loaded with cancer fighting antioxidants. Berries have been shown to increase memory, and are high in fiber, calcium, magnesium, Vitamin C, and Vitamin K.

Mini Onion Quiches • Servings: 10-12

These mini quiches are great to freeze for a quick on the go breakfast later. Here, a typical crust is substituted with shredded coconut.

³/₄ Cup Shredded Coconut
4 Tablespoons Butter, Melted
1 Cup Chopped Green Onion With Tops
2 Tablespoons Butter
2 Eggs
1 Cup Whole Milk
¹/₂ Teaspoon Sea Salt
¹/₄ Teaspoon Pepper
1 Cup Swiss Cheese, Grated

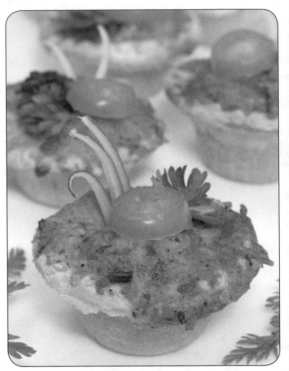

Preheat oven to 300°F. Combine coconut and melted butter. Divide coconut among mini muffin tins. Saute onion for 10 minutes in 2 tablespoons butter.

Cool onions then divide evenly over coconut crust. Beat eggs, add milk, salt, pepper, and swiss cheese. Pour by spoonfuls on top of onions in tins. Do not fill to the top as they will run over. Bake until set, about 15-20 minutes. Do Not Overbake.

Salmon Frittata • Servings: 4

Frittatas make for a beautiful presentation. Experiment with your own favorite ingredients. Pretty much anything goes!

2 Teaspoons Grape Seed Oil
¹/₂ Small Onion, Chopped
1 Small Bunch Asparagus Tops, chopped in small, bite sized pieces
4 Ounces Smoked Wild Salmon, Diced (or use leftover salmon)
6 Eggs
¹/₂ Cup Organic Cream or Half-n-Half
8 Ounces Organic Cream Cheese, softened to room temperature
1 Teaspoon Fresh Dill, Chopped
Sea Salt and Pepper to taste

Heat oven to 375°F. Sauté onion and asparagus in oven proof skillet until slightly tender. Add salmon and heat through. Take pan off heat. In a medium bowl, whisk eggs and cream. Add cream cheese in small chunks, try to blend as much as possible. Don't worry if there are lumps. Pour mix over the salmon and asparagus and add salt and pepper. Stir slowly just to combine ingredients. Cook over medium/low heat until edges look set. Remove from stove and finish cooking in oven for 17 - 20 minutes. Flip over onto serving platter. Garnish with sliced avocado, if desired.

Smoothies

Protein Smoothie
Mint Choco-Nut Dream
Raspberry Explosion
Green Banana Smoothie
Veggie-Berry Smoothie
Tropical Smoothie
Cool-Down Smoothie
Apple-Almond Smoothie
Spicy Cinnamon Smoothie
Salad Smoothie
Super Easy Egg Nog

Smoothies are a terrific start to the day because they are fast, versatile, and healthy. Get creative with your smoothies and don't be afraid to experiment with the ingredients. Always add in some good fats like hemp seeds, hemp seed oil, flax seeds or flaxseed oil, plus extra protein from a raw egg, or extra greens like spinach, kale, or a quality greens powder. Here are a few ideas to get you started.

Protein Smoothie • Servings: 1

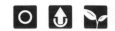

This smoothie uses low glycemic fruit and good fats.

Handful of Frozen Berries
(Strawberries, raspberries, blueberries, blackberries)
Raw Milk or Coconut Milk to taste and desired consistency
1 Scoop Whey Protein

Optional: Add greens like romaine lettuce or spinach and/or add good fats like hemp or flax. Mix everything together in a blender or Vita-Mix®.

Tip: You may add whey or hemp protein for added protein.

Mint Choco-nut Dream • Servings: 1

A breakfast smoothie that really tastes like a dessert!

1-2 Scoops Chocolate Whey Protein Powder
¹/₄ -¹/₂ Can Coconut Milk
1 Tablespoons Mint Flavored Greens Powder
1 Teaspoon Organic Cocoa

¹/₂ - 1 Teaspoon spoonable Stevia
1 Tablespoon Hemp Seed Oil (optional)
1 Teaspoon Almond Butter (optional)

Add water or ice to desired consistency. Mix everything together in a blender or Vita-Mix®.

Raspberry Explosion • Servings: 1

For the raspberry lover

1-2 Scoops Berry-Flavored Whey Protein Powder
3 Tablespoons Full Fat Organic Yogurt
¹/₄ to ¹/₂ Cup Frozen or Fresh Berries
Water to desired consistency
¹/₂ - 1 Teaspoon spoonable Stevia
1 Teaspoon Greens Powder (optional)
1 Teaspoon Hemp Seed Oil (optional)

Mix everything together in a blender or Vita-Mix®.

Green Banana Smoothie • Servings 1

Here is a great way to get that super healthy greens in your body.

1 Banana, Preferably Frozen, Sliced
2 Cups Chopped Kale
1-2 Teaspoons Ground Flaxseed, Optional
1 Teaspoon Stevia
¹/₂ Cup Coconut Milk, Almond Milk or Whole Milk

TIP: Save this one for after exercise because of the high sugar content of the bananas.

Put into a blender or Vita-Mix®. and blend.
Kale may take a while to blend so be patient with it.

Veggie-Berry Smoothie • Servings 2-4

Here is another variation on a kale smoothie.
This gives the added benefit of more fruits and veggies. .

1 Cup Coconut, Almond, or Rice Milk
1 Cup Water
2 Medium Kale Leaves
6 Baby Carrots
8 Fresh Strawberries

1 Cup Frozen Berries
½ Banana
¼ Cup Cranberries, Fresh or Frozen
2 Tablespoons Ground Flaxseed

Put everything in a blender or Vita-Mix®. and blend. It may take a while to blend the kale.

• •

Tropical Smoothie • Servings: 2

2 Cups Organic Green Grapes
1 Large Wedge Pineapple (with core if using a Vita-Mix®.)
2 Cups Fresh Spinach
2-3 Pitted Dates
½ Apple Peeled and Sliced (If using a Vita-Mix®. keep core, seeds, and skin)
2 Cups Ice
Quality Whey Protein (Optional)

Using a Vita-Mix®, blend on High for 45 seconds to 1 minute. If you do not have Vita-Mix®, you may have to skip the pineapple core, apple core and seeds. Enjoy!

• •

Cool-down Smoothie • Servings: 1

You won't believe how good this tastes. Remember to save this type of recipe for right after exercise as the sugar content in the bananas is high.

1 Frozen Banana
1 Handful Baby Spinach, Washed and Trimmed
1 Cup Coconut Milk
½ Teaspoon Mint Flakes

Put everything in the blender and blend until smooth. To make it cold, you can freeze the banana or chill the coconut milk beforehand.

Tip: You may add whey or hemp protein for added protein.

• •

Apple-Almond Smoothie • Servings: 1

Handful of Greens (Swiss Chard, Spinach, Kale)
¼-½ Cup Coconut Milk
1 Frozen Banana, Sliced
Spoonful Almond Butter
1 Apple, Peeled

Put everything in the blender and blend for 30-45 seconds.

Spicy Cinnamon Smoothie • Servings: 1-2

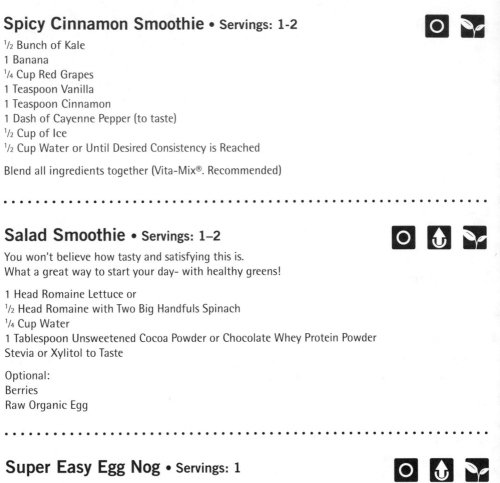

$\frac{1}{2}$ Bunch of Kale
1 Banana
$\frac{1}{4}$ Cup Red Grapes
1 Teaspoon Vanilla
1 Teaspoon Cinnamon
1 Dash of Cayenne Pepper (to taste)
$\frac{1}{2}$ Cup of Ice
$\frac{1}{2}$ Cup Water or Until Desired Consistency is Reached

Blend all ingredients together (Vita-Mix®. Recommended)

· ·

Salad Smoothie • Servings: 1-2

You won't believe how tasty and satisfying this is.
What a great way to start your day- with healthy greens!

1 Head Romaine Lettuce or
$\frac{1}{2}$ Head Romaine with Two Big Handfuls Spinach
$\frac{1}{4}$ Cup Water
1 Tablespoon Unsweetened Cocoa Powder or Chocolate Whey Protein Powder
Stevia or Xylitol to Taste

Optional:
Berries
Raw Organic Egg

· ·

Super Easy Egg Nog • Servings: 1

This is an individual serving size of eggnog. It is quick and easy, healthy,
and a great treat especially during the holidays.

1 Whole Egg
$\frac{1}{4}$ Teaspoon Organic Vanilla
$\frac{1}{4}$ - $\frac{1}{2}$ Teaspoon Stevia or Xylitol, or to Taste
1 Cup Coconut Milk
Nutmeg to Taste
1 Pinch Sea Salt

Beat the egg with the sweetener of your choice along with salt. Pour into a glass. Add vanilla and milk
and stir to mix. Sprinkle a little ground nutmeg on top.

> _Greens_ – This would include kale, chard, spinach, and collards. Kale has the highest
> antioxidant rating of all vegetables, and is therefore a proven fighter and preventer of
> cancer. Greens are high in calcium, iron, Vitamins A, C, and K, betacarotene, fiber, protein,
> and sulfur, which helps the body detoxify. Greens can be mixed into soups and smoothies,
> without any noticable change in taste. Whatever you do, get greens in your diet.

Salads and Slaws

Salads are a must for everyone. Try to eat at least one per day. The options are endless but here are some ideas to get you started. Mix and Match any/all of the following:

• Greens: Romaine, spring mix, spinach, endive, cabbage, etc.

• Nuts/seeds: pumpkin seeds, sunflower seeds, pine nuts, pecans, walnuts, almonds

• Veggies: onions, celery, bell peppers, broccoli, artichokes, tomatoes, olives, peas, cucumbers, mushrooms, asparagus, avocado, kelp powder

• Protein: turkey, chicken, thin sliced beef, hard boiled egg, fish/salmon

• Fruit: blueberries, strawberries, cranberries, apple slices

• Oils: olive oil, avocado oil, mayonnaise

• Acids: vinegar (apple cider, red wine vinegar, white wine vinegar, balsamic), lemon juice, lime juice

• Spices: basil, cilantro, dill, garlic, garlic salt, ginger, parsley, tarragon, pepper, gomasio

Curried Turkey and Rice Salad • Servings: 6

This is a colorful salad that is great warm or chilled. You can use as many or as few ingredients as you want or have on hand. This stores well in the refrigerator for a quick lunch/dinner side.

Salad:
1 Cup Water
2 Tablespoons Curry Powder
1 Teaspoon Garlic, Minced
1/2 Teaspoon Ground Ginger
1/2 Teaspoon Sea Salt
1 Small Onion, Chopped
1 Cup Brown Rice, Toasted Millet, or Bulgar Wheat, Cooked
3/4 Pound Turkey or Chicken, Cooked, Cut Into 1/4 Strips

Optional:
1 Granny Smith Apple, Cut Into 1/2 Inch Cubes
1 Cup Celery, Chopped
1 Cup Red Bell Peppers, Chopped
1/2 Cup Golden Raisins

Vinagrette:
3 Tablespoons Balsamic Vinegar
3 Tablespoons Red Wine Vinegar
2/3 Cup Olive Oil
2 Teaspoons Dijon Mustard
1 Clove Garlic, Crushed

Salt And Pepper To Taste
Optional Toppings:
1/4 Cup Shredded Coconut
1/4 Cup Chopped Nuts

In a large saucepan over high heat, combine the water, curry powder, garlic, ginger, salt and onion. Bring to a boil, remove from heat and stir in rice. Cover and set aside to cool. In a large bowl, combine the turkey, apple, celery, bell pepper, green onion, and raisins. Stir together then stir in cooked rice mixture. To make vinnaigrette: in a small bowl, whisk together the balsamic vinegar, red wine vinegar, oil, mustard, honey, garlic, salt and pepper. Toss salad with vinaigrette. Serve immediatly or cover to refrigerate for 30 to 40 minutes or until well chilled.

TIP: You can serve this on its own or rolled up in lettuce leaves.

Taktouka (Moroccan Cooked Salad) • Servings: 2-4

This is a cooked salad that is often eaten as a dip. Like many other recipes in this book, it can be eaten warm or cold.

2 Ripe Tomatoes, Quartered	3 Tablespoons Olive Oil
1 Small Onion, Chopped	2 Cloves Garlic, Crushed
½ Cucumber, Halved Lengthwise, Seeded, and Chopped	½ Teaspoon Cumin
1 Green Bell Pepper, Halved Seeded And Chopped	2 Tablespoons Cilantro, Chopped
2 Tablespoons Lemon Juice	Sea Salt And Black Pepper

Put the tomatoes, onions, cucumber, and green bell pepper into a pan. Add ¼ cup water and simmer for 5 minutes. Let cool. Combine the lemon juice, olive oil, and garlic, and cumin. Strain the vegetables, then transfer to a bowl. Pour the dressing over them, season with salt and pepper and stir in the chopped cilantro.

TIP: Serve with raw vegetables, flatbread, or flax meal bread .

Raspberry Pecan Summer Salad • Servings 4-6

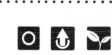

This is a great summertime salad with just the right amount of sweetness.

⅓ Cup Raspberry Spreadable Fruit (No Sugar)
8 Cups Organic Torn Greens
1 Cup Fresh Raspberries
¼ Cup Raspberry Vinegar
¼ Cup Olive Oil
½ Cup Pecans
1 Teaspoon Poppy Seeds
1 Medium Avocado, Chopped
1 Cup Mushroom, Sliced

In a blender combine the spreadable fruit, vinegar, olive oil, and poppy seeds. (or, combine ingredients in a medium bowl and whisk together) In a large salad bowl, combine the greens, raspberries, avocado, mushrooms, and pecans. Drizzle dressing over the salad. Toss to combine.

Chinese Cabbage Salad • Servings: 4-6

This is easy and very good for you. Cabbage is nature's broom and has numerous health benefits.

2 Tablespoons Soy Sauce or Tamari	1 Yellow Bell Pepper, Cut Into Thin Strips
2 Tablespoons Olive Oil	2 Tablespoons Dark Sesame Oil
1 Tablespoon Fresh Ginger, Grated	2 Tablespoons Sesame Seeds, Toasted
1 Small Napa Cabbage, Cut Into Thin Slices	Cooked Chicken (optional)

In a small bowl, mix 2 teaspoons soy sauce or tamari, 1 tablespoon grated ginger, 2 tablespoons dark sesame oil, and 2 tablespoons olive oil. Mix cabbage, bell pepper, add chicken, drizzle with soy sauce or tamari mixture and sprinkle with sesame seeds.

TIP: You can also add cooked chicken, turkey, beef, or hemp seeds for more protein.

Lime and Walnut Coleslaw

A great tangy, crunchy salad. This is a great alternative to mayonnaise based slaws.

1 ½ Cups Raw Walnut Pieces
½ Head Medium-Large Cabbage
1 Basket of Tiny Cherry Tomatoes, Quartered (optional – not pictured here)
1 Jalapeño Pepper, Seeded and Diced
¾ Cup Parsley or Cilantro, Chopped
¼ Cup Freshly Squeezed Lime Juice
2 Tablespoons Olive Oil
¼ Teaspoon Sea Salt

TIP: Leave out the Jalapeño if you like it milder.

Cut the cabbage into two quarters and cut out the core. Using a knife shred each quarter into very thin slices. Cut long pieces in half. Combine the cabbage, walnuts, tomatoes, Jalapeño (optional), and cilantro or parsley in a bowl. In a separate bowl combine the lime juice, olive oil, salt. Add to the cabbage mixture and gently stir.

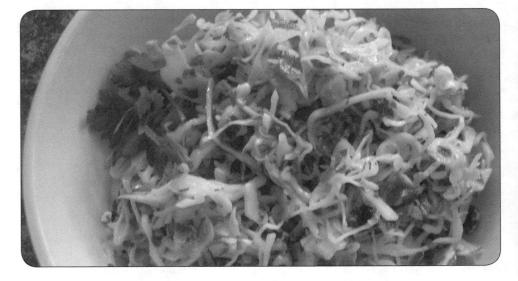

. . . .

Not Tuna Salad

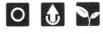

This is both a great meat alternative and a terrific raw food recipe

1 Cup Sunflower Seeds, Soaked 8-12 Hours
1 Cup Almonds Soaked 8-12 Hours
½ Cup Lemon Juice
¼ Cup Minced Celery
2 Teaspoons of Kelp Powder

¼ Cup Minced Red Onion
¼ Cup Minced Parsley
2 Tablespoons Minced Fresh Dill
1 Teaspoon Sea Salt

Process the almonds, sunflower seeds, sea salt, and lemon juice in a food processor until mixture sticks together in a ball. You may need to stop the machine and scrape down the walls with a spatuala. Add the remaining ingredients with your hands. Not Salmon Salad: Add 2 grated carrots to processing mix. (Core Plan only)

Tip: Serve in lettuce wraps, endive leaves, or red bell pepper halves.

Broccoli Cranberry Salad • Servings: 4-6

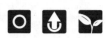

This is a popular recipe that has been improved with better ingredients. It is great for picnics and potlucks.

5 Cups Raw Broccoli Florets, Chopped
½ Cup Red Onion, Chopped
½ Cup Organic Shredded Cheese, Optional
1 Cup Turkey Bacon, Cooked And Crumbled
1 Cup Raw Sunflower Seeds
1 Cup Dried Cranberries

Dressing:
¾ Cup Mayonnaise
stevia or Xylitol to Taste
2 Tablespoons Red Wine Vinegar
¼ Teaspoon Pepper

Combine all salad ingredients in a large mixing bowl; mix well. Combine dressing ingredients in a small mixing bowl. Mix until thoroughly combined using a fork or wire whisk. Add dressing to salad and mix well. Refrigerate 1 hour.

• •

Chicken Artichoke Salad • Servings: 4

A more elegant version of chicken salad, this can be eaten cold or heated.

4 Cups Cooked Chicken Breasts, Chopped
1 (14 Ounces) Can Artichoke Hearts, Drained And Chopped
½ Cup Toasted Pecans, Chopped
½ Cup Mayonnaise
1 Teaspoon Celery Salt
½ Teaspoon Pepper

Stir together all ingredients; cover and chill until ready to serve.

TIP: For a warm version, place on whole wheat bread and bake in the oven at 425°F for 10 minutes. (Core Plan Only)

• •

Taco Salad

Great for families. This recipe allows you to have taco night without needing the taco shells. Spread a variety of toppings on the table and let everyone customize their own.

Basic Chili Recipe	Tomato, chopped
Mixed Lettuces	Red Bell Pepper, Chopped
Spinach	Black Olives, Sliced
Sprouts	Avocados or Guacamole
Black beans, cooked	Salsa

TIP: You can use salsa for dressing or mix salsa with mayonnaise for a creamy salsa dressing.

Mix your salad ingredients and top with the chili.

Soups

> *Soup it Up:* Soup is very versatile, portable, satisfying, and fast. The heat of the soup and the volume of liquid really make the body feel full and satisfied. It is even used in many countries to detox the body. Soups are a great way to add vegetables to your diet which you may not eat otherwise: cabbage blended into soup adds a lot of nutrition, but does not alter the taste of the soup considerably. Be wary of canned soups, pre-made soups, and restaurant soups, which often hide tons table salt, fat, MSG, and other artificial ingredients. You are much better off making it yourself.

Butternut Squash and Leek Soup • Servings: 4-6

Even if you think you don't like squash, this is a delicious soup. It is very creamy without the use of milk or cream. This one takes a little bit of preparation to roast the garlic and cook the squash but that can be done ahead of time.

1 Head of Garlic, Roasted, See Below	2 Cups Water
4 Teaspoons Olive Oil	2 Cup Organic Chicken Broth
6 Large Leeks, Thinly Sliced	¹/₂ Teaspoon Sea Salt
4 Cup Butternut Squash, Baked	¹/₂ Teaspoon Black Pepper, Ground

Preheat oven to 350°F. Cut squash in half and brush with some olive oil. Place cut side down on a baking dish and bake for about 30-40 minutes or until squash is soft. Scoop out squash and set aside. Remove the white papery skin from garlic head but do not peel or separate the cloves. Wrap head in foil. Bake at 350°F for 1 hour; cool 10 minutes. Separate cloves; squeeze to extract garlic pulp. Discard skins. Heat oil in a large saucepan over medium-high heat. Add leek; sauté 5 minutes or until tender.

Stir in garlic, squash, 2 cups water, broth, salt, and pepper; bring to a boil. Reduce heat, and simmer until well mixed. Place half the squash mixture in a blender. (if the mixture is still hot you may need to remove the center piece of the blender lid to let steam escape- if so cover with a towel instead.) Blend until smooth. Repeat procedure with remaining squash mixture. Do not overcrowd your blender with hot foods!

Chicken Sausage Soup • Servings: 4-6

Please watch ingredients for sausage- some chicken/turkey sausage contains dangerous additives like nitrites and some will have pork casings. Read your labels or ask at the meat counter.

1 Quart Organic Chicken Broth
1 Quart Water
6-8 Chicken or Turkey Sausage Links
3 Cloves Garlic, Sliced
1 Medium Onion, Chopped
2-3 Heads Escarole or Spinach
1 Can Cannelloni Beans (White Beans), Drained
Fresh Parsley
Lemon Zest

Brown the onion and garlic in a small amount of olive oil in a medium sized stock pot. Add chicken stock and water along with salt to taste. Bring to a boil and simmer. In the meantime, brown chicken sausages in a separate frying pan and cut into chunks. Set aside. Add chopped escarole or spinach and canneloni beans to the stock mixture. Let simmer for 5-10 minutes. Add the sausage back in right before serving. Top with fresh parsley and lemon zest.

Cream of Cauliflower Soup • Servings: 4-6

Most white foods are typically on the unhealthy list but cauliflower is the exception. Even kids will love this creamy white soup.

2 Cups Cauliflower, Chopped
1 Can Coconut Milk
1/2 Cup Celery, Chopped
1/2 Cup Onion, Chopped
1 Teaspoon Sea Salt
1/8 Teaspoon Black Pepper
1/4 Teaspoon Curry Powder
2 Tablespoons Butter
2 Tablespoons Coconut Flour
1 Cup Water

Simmer cauliflower, celery, and onion together in water for 20 minutes or until very tender. Drain and add back in 1 cup of water. Puree, a little at a time, in a blender at low speed. (Do not overcrowd the blender with hot foods). Heat butter in a saucepan over medium heat; blend in flour and cook until blended, stirring frequently. Add coconut milk slowly and stir until smooth. Mix in puree, salt, pepper, and curry powder, stirring occasionally until hot but do not boil.

. . . .

Italian Spinach Soup • Servings: 4-6

Also called Italian Wedding Soup, this is a great soup for all year round.

Meatballs:
1 Egg
1/2 Cup Parmesan Cheese
1 Small Onion
1 Teaspoon Sea Salt
1/2 Teaspoon Pepper
1 Teaspoon Garlic Powder
2 Pounds Ground Turkey
2 Tablespoons Coconut Oil

Soup:
1 Quart Organic Chicken Broth
1 Cup Spinach, Chopped
1 Teaspoon Onion Powder
1 Tablespoon Chopped Parsley
1 Teaspoon Sea Salt
1/2 Teaspoon Pepper
1/2 Teaspoon Garlic Powder

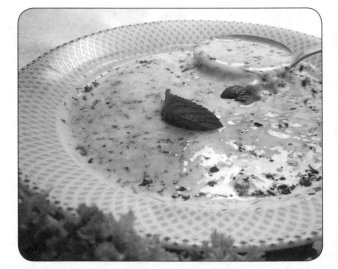

Meatballs: In a bowl, combine all meatball ingredients. Shape into 1 inch balls. Fry in coconut oil until done. Set aside. Mix other ingredients in a saucepan and bring to a boil. When spinach is wilted, add the meatballs back in and serve.

TIP: If you want to use this soup over a few days, leave the spinach out until you are ready to reheat it then add it into the broth as it heats.
TIP: The meatballs do not contain breadcrumbs so they are a little more fragile. Fry them with care or bake in the oven.

Quick French Onion Soup • Servings: 4-6

This is a classic favorite that you can duplicate in record time. It is a great start to a meal.

1 Tablespoon of Coconut Oil
3 Cloves Garlic, Minced
3 Medium Onions, Sliced Into Rings
1 Pound Button Mushrooms, Brushed And Sliced
1 Tablespoon Dried Thyme Leaves

2 Teaspoons Dried Marjoram Leaves
¼ Cup Tamari or Liquid Aminos
2 Quarts Filtered Water or Organic Chicken Stock
Slices of Raw Swiss or Provolone Cheese, Optional

In a large skillet over medium heat, melt oil. Add garlic and onions, and cook for a few minutes until translucent. Add mushrooms and cook, stirring frequently, until mushrooms are tender 2-3 more minutes. Stir in thyme, marjoram leaves and 1 Tablespoon tamari. Sauté a few seconds more to let flavors develop. Add water and bring soup back to the boiling point. Reduce heat and simmer 5 more minutes. Add remaining tamari. If desired, put soup in oven safe bowls and add shredded cheese on top. Put on a baking tray and broil until cheese is melted and bubbly.

Chilled Cream of Tomato Soup • Servings: 2-4

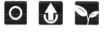

Cold soups are great for hot summer days or for packing in a portable lunch. This raw food soup is full of valuable nutrients.

3 Ripe Tomatoes, Seeded and Chopped (about 1½ cups)
¼ Cup Water
½ Teaspoon Crushed Garlic (1 clove)
¼ Teaspoon Onion Powder

¼ Teaspoon Sea Salt
½ Ripe Avocado, Chopped
1 Tablespoons Extra Virgin Olive Oil
2 Teaspoon Minced Fresh Dill Weed or Basil

Place the tomatoes, water, garlic, onion powder, and salt in a blender and process until smooth. Add avocado and olive oil and blend again until smooth. Add the dill weed and blend briefly, just to mix. Serve immediately or chill in refrigerator.

Cream of Zucchini Soup • Servings: 2-4

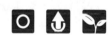

This soup is creamy and delicious without the use of milk or cream. The taste is very exotic but simple.

1 Cup Water, Plus Additional Water to Thin
2 Medium Zucchini, Peeled and Chopped (About 2 Cups)
2 Stalks Celery, Chopped
2 Tablespoons Lemon Juice
2 Tablespoons Extra Virgin Olive Oil
2 Tablespoons Minced Fresh Dill (or 2 Teaspoons Dried)
2 Teaspoons Mellow White Miso
2 Small Cloves, Crushed

½ Teaspoon Sea Salt, or to Taste
Dash Cayenne

1 Avocado, Mashed Place the water, zucchini, celery, lemon juice, olive oil, miso, garlic, salt and cayenne in a blender or Vita-Mix® and process until smooth. Add the avocado and dill and blend briefly. Add additional water to thin the soup to desired consistency, and blend. Serve chilled or at room temperature. Store in a sealed container in the refrigerator, Cream of Zucchini Soup will keep up to three days. This creamy soup is delicious served chilled at room temperature, or warmed gently on the stove or in the dehydrator.

Breads

Apple Flaxseed Muffins • Servings: 8-12

Most muffins are loaded with sugar, bad fats, and refined flours. This healthy version is both satisfying and delicious

1¼ Cup Flaxseed Meal
2 Teaspoons Aluminum Free Baking Powder
1 Tablespoon Cinnamon
1 Teaspoon Nutmeg
½ Teaspoon Sea Salt
Stevia or Xylitol or Equivalent Equal to 2/3 Cup Sugar
4 Large Eggs, Beaten
¼ Cup Olive Oil
½ Cup Water
1 Tablespoon Pure Vanilla (No Sugar – Check the Ingredients)
1 Medium Granny Smith Apple, Chopped Fairly Finely or Grated
½ Cup Chopped Pecans (Optional)

Note: You can also add any type of berries to the batter.

Tip: These muffins will look somewhat spongy inside.

Preheat oven to 350 F. Prepare a muffin tin with silicone baking cups or paper liners.
Mix the dry ingredients together. Mix the wet ingredients. Add the wet to the dry and combine thoroughly. Let batter stand 10 minutes. Separate batter into the muffin pan and bake for approximately 18 minutes, or until a toothpick comes out clean.

• •

Flax Meal Bread • Servings: 1 Loaf

Staying away from refined carbohydrates like bread is often difficult because they are a common staple in most people's diet. This is a healthy, crunchy alternative.

2 Cups Flaxseed Meal
1 Tablespoon Aluminum Free Baking Powder
1 Teaspoon Sea Salt
Stevia and/or Xylitol Equivalent to 1-2 Tablespoons Sugar
5 Beaten Eggs
½ Cup Water
⅓ Cup Grapeseed or Coconut Oil

Preheat oven to 350 F. Prepare pan or a half-sheet pan with parchment paper or a silicone mat.
Mix dry ingredients - a whisk works well. Mix wet ingredients; add to dry combining well. Let batter set for 2 to 3 minutes to thicken up. Pour batter onto pan. Bake for about 20 minutes, until it springs back when you touch the top and/or is visibly browning.
Cool and cut into whatever size slices you desire.

> *Olive Oil – Olive oil is used extensively in Mediterranean diets which are very healthy. Olive oil is high in phenols (antioxidants), monounsaturated fats, and oleic acid. Olive oil has been shown to help optimize cholesterol ratios, lower blood pressure, and prevent cancer. The purest form and least processed is Extra Virgin Olive Oil. To prevent oxidation and rancidity, olive oil should not be heated beyond its low smoke point. It is best used on salads or sprinkled on foods after they are cooked.*

Pizza Crust/Flat Bread • Servings: 1 Pizza Crust

This is a great substitute for regular pizza crust. It makes a nice crispy crust rather than a soft doughy one. Use it in place of crackers as well.

1 Tablespoon Gluten Free Dry Yeast
1½ Cups Almond Flour
1 Cup Garbanzo Bean Flour
2 Tablespoons Dry Milk Powder
2 Teaspoons Xanthan Gum
½ Teaspoon Sea Salt
1 Teaspoon Unflavored Gelatin Powder
1 Teaspoon Italian Herb Seasoning
⅔ Cup Warm Water
1 Teaspoon Olive Oil
1 Teaspoon Organic Apple Cider Vinegar
Grapeseed Oil

Preheat oven to 425°F. In a medium bowl, mix the yeast, flours, dry milk powder, xanthan gum, salt, gelatin powder, and Italian herb seasoning. Use an electric mixer on low speed to blend dry ingredients. Add warm water, olive oil, and vinegar. Mix on high for three minutes. The dough will be very sticky.

Coat or spray a pan with grapeseed oil. Place the dough on the pan. Sprinkle some bean flour on the dough to help press it evenly into the pan. (12" round or 9" x 13") Bake for 10 minutes. Remove the pizza crust from the oven and cut into pieces to eat or top with your favorite sauce and toppings. Bake for an additional 15-20 minutes.

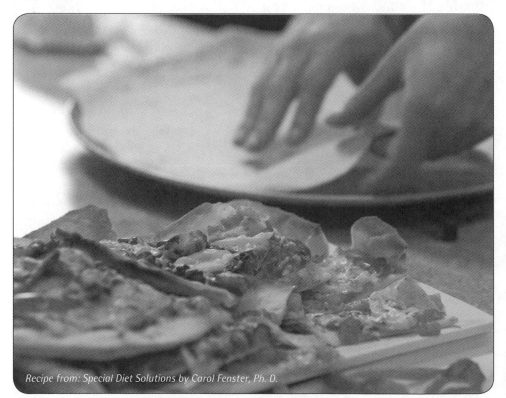

Recipe from: Special Diet Solutions by Carol Fenster, Ph. D.

Flax Crackers • Servings: 16 crackers

A crunchy, nutritious, and tasty snack. Good with dips, spreads, or just by themselves.

1 Cup Flaxseed Meal
1½ Teaspoon Garlic Powder
½ Teaspoon Salt
½ Cup Water
¼ - ⅓ Cup Parmesan Cheese, Grated (Optional)

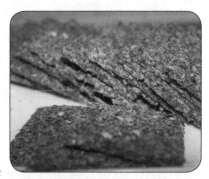

Heat oven to 400° F. Mix all ingredients together. Spoon onto sheet pan which is covered with lightly greased parchment paper. Cover with another piece of parchment or waxed paper. Roll out the mixture to about ⅛ inch trying to keep it even all the way across. Remove the paper and push any thinned out edges towards the middle so they don't cook before the center. Bake until the center is no longer soft, about 15-18 minutes. Do not let it brown around the edges. Let cool completely. Cut into pieces with a pizza cutter or just break into pieces.

Tip. Feel free to experiment with the spices in this recipe. You can use chili powder, cumin, Italian herbs, curry powder, tumeric, sesame seeds, onion powder, crushed red pepper, kelp powder, etc.

Almond Cookies • Servings: about 15 cookies

This is a quick, tasty treat with no flour making it advanced plan approved.

½ Teaspoon Baking Soda
1 Teaspoon Vanilla Extract
⅛-¼ Cup Xylitol
1 Cup Almond Meal
1 Egg
½ Teaspoon Grated Lemon Peel

Preheat oven to 350°F and grease cookie sheet with grapeseed oil. Stir together almond meal, Xylitol and baking soda In a medium bowl. Add beaten egg and vanilla extract and mix well. Shape dough into balls one inch apart on cookie sheet. Bake until puffed and golden, about 10 minutes. Cool cookies on baking sheet about 2 minutes before transferring to a rack or waxed paper to cool.

TIP: For another variation, drizzle with melted unsweetened chocolate with stevia or Xylitol added to taste.

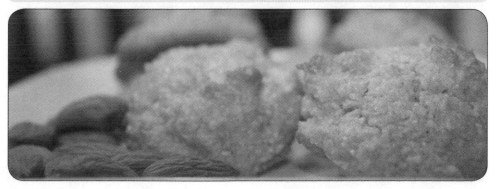

Entrees

Beef Stew

Meatloaf

Grilled Steak with Chimichurri Sauce

Basic Chili

Stuffed Peppers

Lemon Lamb

Asian Turkey Lettuce Wraps

Chicken Asparagus Marsala

Chicken Cacciatore

Endless Chicken Salad

Orange Chicken

Tex-Mex Skillet

Chicken Savoy

Grilled Chicken with Chili Pepper,
Bok Choy, and Ginger

Carribean Chicken

Holiday Roast Turkey

Marinated Chicken Satay

Buffalo Chicken Rolls

Easy Cuban Style Chicken Breasts

Fish Fry Dinner

Fancy Salmon

Teriyaki Salmon

Crispy Salmon Cakes with
Red Pepper and Tomato Sauce

Smoked Salmon Tartar

Roasted Vegetable Lasagna

Stuffed Porto Patty

Beef Stew • Servings: 4

This is a perfect example of taking a traditional favorite and making it super healthy.

2 Tablespoons Coconut Oil
1 Pound Grass Fed Beef Round or Stew Meat, Chopped Into 1" Cubes
1 Teaspoon Salt
$\frac{1}{2}$ Teaspoon Ground Pepper
$\frac{3}{4}$ Cup Onion, Chopped
3 Cloves Garlic, Chopped
2 Tablespoons Tomato Paste
2 Tablespoons Worcestershire Sauce

4 Stalks Celery, Sliced
1 Pound Mushrooms
3 Cups Filtered Water
3 Cups Organic Beef Broth
$\frac{1}{2}$ Cup Parsley, Chopped
1 Tablespoon Thyme
1 Bay Leaf

Heat a large stockpot to medium high heat. While heating, sprinkle beef with salt and pepper. Add oil and sauté beef, stirring frequently, for 7-9 minutes until browned. Remove beef pieces from pot. Add onions, garlic, bay leaves, and thyme to pot and sauté until translucent or simply put them into a crockpot with the juices from the browning pot. Stir in tomato paste and Worcestershire sauce. Add celery, and mushrooms. Stir to coat and sauté a few more minutes. Add browned beef, water, and stock. Reduce to low and simmer covered for several hours, until beef is tender. Serve sprinkled with parsley.

TIP: Using a crockpot for this recipe allows you to have a fresh, healthy meal when you get home. You can even brown the meat the night before so preparation time in the morning is only a few minutes.

Meatloaf • Servings: 4

Here is another traditional favorite that everyone will love.

1 Pound Grass Fed Ground Beef
1 Small Yellow Onion, Chopped
1 Clove Garlic, Minced
$\frac{1}{2}$ Cup Flat Leaf Parsley, Finely Chopped
1 Large Egg, Lightly Beaten
1 Cup Sprouted Grain Bread, Lightly Toasted and Processed into Crumbs
$\frac{2}{3}$ Cup Organic Tomato Paste, or Fruit Sweetened Ketchup (no sugar), Divided
1 Teaspoon Sea Salt
$\frac{1}{2}$ Teaspoon Pepper

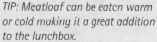

TIP: Meatloaf can be eaten warm or cold making it a great addition to the lunchbox.

Preheat oven to 375°F. In a medium bowl, combine chopped onion, garlic, parsley, egg, and $\frac{1}{3}$ cup ketchup. Add breadcrumbs and beef. Season with salt and pepper. Mix until well combined. Place mixture in a 6 cup capacity loaf pan (8 x 4 inch) or simply shape into a loaf in a glass baking dish. Pat gently to make a rounded top. Do not pack. Bake meatloaf 50 minutes. Remove from oven; brush with remaining 1/3 cup tomato paste or ketchup . Return to the oven; Bake until an instant-read thermometer inserted into the center of the loaf reads 160°F, approximately 10 - 20 minutes. Cool meat loaf for 10 minutes in pan before slicing.

Grass Fed Beef – Cows were meant to roam pastures and eat grass, NOT grain. In changing the cow's diet to cheap grains, its meat has become far less healthy. Grain feeding cows would ultimately kill them by acidosis, if they were not first slaughtered. On the other hand, grass fed beef has 60% more Omega-3 fatty acids, and the ideal ratio of Omega-6 to Omega-3 which is most important in disease prevention. Grass fed beef is high in iron, Vitamin B12, monounsaturated fat, and zinc.

Grilled Steak With Chimichurri Sauce • Servings: 2

Grass fed beef with this spicy green sauce is a real taste treat. It is so easy to make you will be in and out of the kitchen very quickly.

³/₄ Cup Finely Chopped Fresh Italian Parsley
¹/₂ Cup Olive Oil
3 Tablespoons Fresh Lemon Juice
2¹/₂ Tablespoons Finely Chopped Garlic
2¹/₂ Teaspoons Dried Crushed Red Pepper
2 Grass-Fed Beef Tenderloin Steaks, 4 to 6 Ounces Each (About 1 Inch Thick)

Place all ingredients (except steak) in a food processor. Pulse until a smooth sauce is achieved. Refrigerate if time permits. (Can be made one day ahead.) Bring to room temperature before using. Sprinkle both sides of steaks with salt and pepper. Place steaks on hot grill pan or barbeque grill and cook until desired wellness, about 3 minutes per side for medium-rare. Slice steaks crosswise and arrange on a platter. Spoon chimichurri sauce over the steaks and serve.

> *Grass-fed meats and free-range chickens have the good fats in the right ratios, unlike store bought meats*

Basic Chili • Servings: 4-6

Everyone should have this recipe in their collection. It is healthy, easy to make, and travels well. You can also use this recipe to make a taco salad. Just put over greens with your favorite toppings.

1 Tablespoon Coconut Oil
¹/₂ Cup Onion, Chopped or Grated
¹/₂ Cup Celery, Chopped
2 Cloves Garlic, Minced
1 Cup Green Pepper, Chopped
1 Can Kidney Beans or Black Beans
2 Teaspoons Oregano
2 Teaspoons Chili Powder
2 Teaspoons Ground Cumin
1 Teaspoon Sea Salt
1 8 Ounce Can Organic Crushed-Tomatoes
1 - 1¹/₂ Pounds Ground Bison, Grass Fed Beef,
  or Ground Turkey

Optional: 1-12 Ounce Jar Prepared Salsa or Pasta sauce (check ingredients) This can be in addition to or to replace the tomatoes (depending on your consistency preference).

In a large skillet melt oil and sauté onions, celery, garlic, and peppers until onion is translucent, 3-4 minutes. Add ground meat, oregano, chili powder, and cumin, continue cooking, stirring frequently, for 5-6 minutes. Pour salt, tomatoes, and salsa, if desired, into pot. Cover, reduce heat and simmer for a minimum of 1 hour for best flavor.

> *TIP: You can use a crockpot for this recipe making preparation even simpler.*
> *TIP: If you are on the Advanced Plan, you can leave out the beans.*

Stuffed Peppers • Servings: 6

A fancy presentation already in individual servings.

6 Whole Bell Peppers, Red, Yellow or Orange Preferred
1 Pound Grass Fed Ground Beef
1 Cup Brown Rice
1 Can Crushed Tomatoes
1 Can Chicken Stock
1 Garlic Clove, Minced
Coarse Sea Salt and Freshly Ground Black Pepper

Preheat oven to 350°F. Season the meat with salt and pepper and brown in skillet on medium-high. In the meantime, cook the rice with half the amount of liquid (using chicken stock rather than water will add flavor) and half the time as noted on the directions. Once the rice mixture is transferred to the peppers, the liquid in the peppers will continue the rice in the oven. Be careful not to overcook the rice. Add the can of tomatoes, including liquid, into the skillet with the ground beef. Once the rice is done, add that to the skillet along with the minced garlic and salt and pepper. Combine all ingredients well.

Cut the tops off the peppers and remove all the seeds from inside. Take your meat and rice mixture and fill the peppers to the top and put the tops back on. Cover the entire baking dish with aluminum foil trying to make sure it doesn't touch the peppers and bake in the oven for about 50 minutes. Remove the foil and cook for an additional 10 minutes. Make sure the peppers are tender, but not falling apart.

TIP: Serve with some freshly grated parmesan cheese.

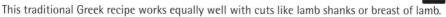

Lemon Lamb • Servings: 6

This traditional Greek recipe works equally well with cuts like lamb shanks or breast of lamb.

¹/₃ Cup Lemon Juice, Freshly Squeezed
3 Pounds Lamb Shanks (or Other Lamb)
1 Tablespoon Olive Oil
2 Cloves Garlic, Crushed
1 Tablespoon Fresh Oregano (Divided) or 2 Teaspoons Dried Oregano (Divided)

Trim skin and all excess fat from the lamb. Cut the meat down the center so that it lays flat and rub both inside and outside surfaces with some of the lemon juice and sprinkle them with salt and pepper. On the inside surface of the meat, sprinkle a teaspoon of dried oregano or ¹/₂ a tablespoon of chopped fresh oregano. Roll the meat up and tie securely.

Heat a tablespoon of olive oil in a pot large enough to take the roll comfortably and brown the meat on all sides. Turn the heat down to low and add to the pot the rest of the lemon juice, the garlic, and another teaspoon of dried oregano or 1 tablespoon of fresh. Cover the pot and simmer very gently, turning occasionally, for about 2¹/₂ hours, till very tender.
To serve, remove the string, slice the meat and pour the lemony juices over the meat.

TIP: If you use a fattier cut, make the dish a day ahead, refrigerate it and remove the fat that coagulates on top. The dish gains even more flavor when made ahead.

Asian Turkey Lettuce Wraps • Servings: 4-5

This is a very tasty dish that will rival any Chinese takeout or elegant Chinese restaurant. It makes a nice presentation for an appetizer as well.

$^1/_2$ Cup Water
3 Tablespoons Organic Almond/Cashew Butter
1 Pound Ground Turkey
1 Tablespoon Sesame Oil
1 Cup Shiitake Mushroom Caps, Chopped
1 Tablespoon Rice Vinegar
1 (8 Ounces) Can Water Chestnuts, Drained and Chopped
3 Cloves Garlic
2 Tablespoons Fresh Ginger, Minced
$^1/_3$ Cup Tamari
$^1/_2$ Cup Green Onions, Optional,
1 Head Lettuce, Separated into Leaves

Cook turkey in skillet about 5 minutes, stirring until turkey crumbles and is no longer pink. Add mushrooms, and next 5 ingredients. Increase heat to medium-high, and cook, stirring constantly, 4 minutes. Add green onions if desired and cook, stirring constantly, 1 minute. Spoon mixture evenly onto lettuce leaves; roll up. Serve with extra tamari sauce if desired.

> *TIP: You can replace the lettuce with all natural whole wheat tortillas as well for the core plan.*
> *TIP: You can also add $^1/_4$ cup chopped carrots that have been lightly steamed for the Core Plan*

Chicken Asparagus Marsala • Servings: 4

Asparagus always give a dish an elegant flair. Here, it also adds beautiful color.

4 Chicken Breast Halves, Boned and Skinned
10 Ounces Asparagus Spears, Cut
2 Tablespoons Butter
1 Tablespoon Coconut or Grapeseed Oil
$^1/_2$ Teaspoon Salt
$^1/_4$ Cup Water
$^1/_8$ Teaspoon Pepper
1 Tablespoon Parsley, Chopped Diagonally into Pieces

$^1/_2$ Pound Mushrooms
$^1/_4$ Cup Marsala Wine

Pound the chicken pieces to $^1/_4$-inch thickness. Melt the butter in a frying pan over medium-high temperature. Add chicken and cook, turning, for about 5 minutes or until the chicken is brown. Remove chicken and set aside. To the drippings remaining in the fry pan, add the asparagus and mushrooms and cook, stirring, for about 3 minutes. Return the chicken to the pan, add the marsala wine, water, salt, and pepper.

Bring the mixture to a boil for 2 minutes to reduce the liquid. Reduce heat, cover and simmer for about 3 minutes or until the chicken and vegetables are tender. Arrange the chicken on a serving platter. Spoon the vegetable sauce over the chicken. Sprinkle with chopped parsley and serve.

> *TIP: The alcohol in the wine will burn off during cooking but make sure you are using a quality Marsala to get the best flavor. If the asparagus is very thick, rather than wasting the tough ends, use a vegetable peeler to peel off the hard outer edge and leave the soft middle intact.*

Chicken Cacciatore • Servings: 4

This is a classic dish that is sure to be part of your regular menu rotations.

2 Pounds Chicken Pieces
1 Medium Onion, Sliced
1/2 Medium Green Pepper, Chopped
1/4 Cup Olive Oil
1 Garlic
1 Can Plum Tomatoes (16 Ounces)

1 Tbl Parsley, Chopped
1/2 Teaspoon Oregano, Crushed
1/4 Teaspoon Thyme
3/4 Teaspoon Salt
1/4 Teaspoon Pepper
1/4 Pound Mushroom, Sliced

TIP: You can modify this recipe by using skinless, boneless chicken breasts.

Heat oil in large skillet. Add chicken pieces, brown and set aside. Add onion, green pepper and garlic. Cook until onion is tender. Force Italian plum tomatoes through a strainer to remove seeds. Add tomato liquid, parsley, oregano, thyme, salt and pepper to skillet. Cook over low heat for 15 minutes; stir occasionally. Add chicken; cover and cook over low heat 45 minutes. Stir occasionally. Add mushrooms. Cook uncovered 15 minutes or until sauce is desired consistency.

· ·

Endless Chicken Salad • Servings: 4

This recipe is so versatile and will get you compliments every time you make it.

4 Chicken Breasts, Cooked and Shredded or Chopped
1/2 - 2/3 Cup Mayonnaise (See Recipe OR Store Bought Mayonnaise Substitute- Check Ingredients)
2 Teaspoons Fresh Lemon Juice
Choose Your Favorites:

Core Plan Add-Ins:
Shredded Carrots
Chopped Apples
Chopped Grapes
Dried Cranberries
Raisins
Mustard

TIP: Serve on a lettuce leaf, on a whole wheat wrap, or whole wheat bread.

TIP: You can also make this into a chicken salad casserole by putting everything in a glass dish, sprinkle with gomasio or finely chopped nuts and heat in a 350 degree oven for 15-18 minutes.

Core and Advanced Add-Ins:
Curry Powder
Gomasio
Chopped Celery
Chopped Pickles
Raw Pecans, Chopped
Raw Walnuts, Chopped
Raw Almonds, Sliced or Slivered

Mix any of the above ingredients with the chicken, mayonnaise and lemon juice.

Nuts - Nuts are great because they have so many health benefits yet they are delicious and offer a great, portable snack option. Nuts have been shown to lower heart disease, prevent cancer, and lower cholesterol. They are loaded with protein, good fats, fiber, magnesium, and antioxidants. The heating and roasting process diminishes some of their nutritional value, therefore they are best raw -- and even better soaked overnight in water.

Orange Chicken • Servings: 4

This is a quick, simple dish with great flavor.

4 Skinless, Boneless Chicken Breasts
2 Teaspoons Olive Oil
2 Teaspoons Butter
¼ Teaspoon Salt

½ Cup White Wine
¼ Teaspoon Freshly Ground Black Pepper
½ Cup Fresh Orange Juice (about 2 Oranges)
⅓ Cups Whole Wheat Flour or Coconut Flour

Place each chicken breast half between pieces of waxed or parchment paper. Pound each piece into ½ inch thickness using a meat mallet or heavy skillet. Sprinkle both sides of chicken evenly with salt and pepper; dredge chicken in flour. Heat oil and butter in a large skillet over medium-high heat; cook for 1 minute or until lightly browned, stirring occasionally. Add chicken to pan; cook 4 minutes on each side or until done. Remove chicken, slice thinly, and keep warm. Add wine and orange juice to pan; cook until reduced and alcohol is burned off to 1/2 cup (about 4 minutes). Serve sauce over chicken.

• •

Tex-Mex Skillet • Servings: 4

Just add everything to one pan and make cleanup a breeze.

1 Pound. Ground Free-range Turkey
1 Pound Ground Grass-fed Beef
2 Tablespoons Grape Seed Oil
1 Small Onion, Diced
3 Cloves Garlic, Minced
1 Bell Pepper, Chopped
1 Tablespoon Ground Cumin
1 Teaspoon Paprika
1 Teaspoon Crushed Red Pepper

½ Jalapeño Pepper (Omit Seeds for Less Heat)
1 Can Chopped Tomatoes, Drained
1 Can Black Beans, Rinsed and drained
Spinach Leaves
Salt and pepper to Taste
Plain Greek Yogurt
1 Avocado, Sliced
1 Tablespoon Fresh Cilantro, Chopped

Sauté onion, bell pepper and garlic in oil for three minutes. Add ground turkey and beef and cook until meat is no longer pink. Add seasonings and stir to heat flavors together. Add tomatoes, black beans, cook on medium heat for 7 minutes. Serve over bed of fresh spinach leaves. Top with dollop of yogurt, avocado slices and fresh cilantro. Option: serve in whole wheat or rye tortilla wrap. (Core Plan Only)

• •

Chicken Savoy • Servings: 4

This chicken is juicy and delectable plus simple to prepare.

4 Boneless Skinless Chicken Breasts
⅛ Cup Extra Virgin Olive Oil
⅔ Cup Water with 1 Tablespoon Sea Salt
2 or 3 Cloves of Garlic, Minced or Grated
½ to 1 Teaspoon Dried Oregano or Basil

Sea and Pepper to Taste
¼ Cup Grated Italian Romano Cheese
3 Tablespoons Balsamic Vinegar

Preheat oven to 450°F. Place the chicken breasts in a 9 x 13 or other shallow baking dish. Cover the chicken with a mixture made of the water, salt, and olive oil. Grate or mince the garlic and sprinkle it on the chicken breasts. Sprinkle the salt, pepper, and other seasoning over the chicken. Sprinkle the Romano cheese over the chicken. Bake at 450°F for 20 to 30 minutes, or until chicken is cooked through. Remove the dish from the oven, and pour off the excess fluid, leaving the chicken in the baking dish. Drizzle with the balsamic vinegar and serve.

Grilled Chicken with Chili Pepper, Bok Choy, and Ginger
• Servings: 2-4

Bok Choy is a type of cabbage that offers tremendous health benefits.
As the main ingredient in this dish, you are receiving maximum nutrition.

1 Cup Organic Chicken Breast
2 Cloves Fresh Garlic, Crushed
1 Tablespoon Fresh Ginger, Grated
1-2 Tablespoons Soy Sauce or Tamari (plus extra for serving)
1 Tablespoon Mirin
2 Cups Bok Choy, Sliced
2 Tablespoons Coconut Oil
2 Cups Fresh Shitake or Portobello Mushrooms, Washed and Sliced
$\frac{1}{2}$ Mild Chili Pepper, Seeded and Chopped
2 Small Green Onions, Sliced
1-2 Teaspoons Dark Sesame Oil (optional)
$\frac{1}{2}$ - 1 Teaspoon Toasted Sesame Seeds

Mix chicken together with half the garlic, half the ginger, soy sauce or tamari, and mirin and set aside. Heat 1 Tablespoon oil in a wok or large pot and add mushrooms, bok choy, chili pepper, green onions and remaining garlic and ginger. Stir fry for about 6 minutes or until bok choy is tender but still crisp. Meanwhile, brush chicken with marinade. Pick up a piece of chicken and let excess juices run off. Place the chicken on the hot grill pan and repeat with remaining chicken. Cook for 2-3 minutes until it is seared and has brown stripes then flip pieces over to cook the other side. Add any remaining marinade to the bok choy mixture, stir, and season with sea salt and pepper, sesame oil, and a dash of soy sauce or tamari. To serve, sprinkle with sesame seeds.

• •

Caribbean Chicken • Servings: 4

This is a recipe that you will be sure to make often because it uses common ingredients. It is hard to believe something so good is so easy.

2 Tablespoon Olive Oil
Coarse Salt and Freshly Ground Pepper
1 Small Onion, Finely Chopped
2 Cloves Garlic, Finely Chopped
$\frac{1}{2}$ Cup Coconut Milk
1 Can (14 ounces) Crushed Tomatoes
2 Pinch Ground Cinnamon
4 Boneless Chicken Breast Halves, Cut into Chunks
2 Tablespoons Curry Powder
Cilantro Leaves, Coarsely Chopped, for Garnish

Heat oil in a large skillet over medium-high heat. Add onions and garlic and cook, stirring, until golden brown. Add tomatoes, chicken, and sprinkle curry powder; season with salt and pepper. Reduce heat to low, and cook, stirring, until mixture has thickened and chicken is cooked through, 15 to 25 minutes. Add coconut milk and stir until well combined; cook 5 minutes more. Sprinkle with cinnamon. Garnish with cilantro and serve immediately.

TIP: This dish is great served with sautéed greens.

Holiday Roast Turkey • Servings: 6-8

This is a fail-proof way of cooking a turkey. It comes out golden on the outside and juicy and moist on the inside.

1 Organic Turkey
$^1/_2$ Pound Butter
$^1/_2$ Teaspoon Dried Sage

$^1/_2$ Teaspoon Dried Thyme
$^1/_2$ Teaspoon Dried Marjoram Leaves
$^1/_2$ Teaspoon Crushed Rosemary

Preheat oven to 425°F. Rinse the turkey inside and out then pat dry, stuff (if desired), and truss. Cut a piece of cheesecloth to a length that will cover the turkey and unfold to a single thickness. Melt $^1/_2$ pound of butter in a small saucepan and add $^1/_2$ teaspoon each of dried sage, thyme, marjoram, and crushed rosemary. Place cheesecloth in the pan and completely saturate. (You can also brush skin with herbed olive oil and baste every 15 minutes.)

Place turkey in oven and reduce heat to 325°F. After 15 minutes, drape butter-soaked cheesecloth over the turkey so that it is completely covered. After an hour, baste the turkey every 15 minutes or so to keep the cheesecloth moist (you can use your leftover butter as well). Remove the cheesecloth for the last 30 minutes of cooking time for crisp skin. Allow the turkey to sit for at least 20 minutes before carving

Marinated Chicken Satay • Servings: 4-6

This is a great speedy dinner. Kids love them because they can eat them right off the sticks.

2 Tablespoons Almond or Cashew Butter
$^1/_2$ Cup Tamari or Soy Sauce
$^1/_2$ Cup Lemon or Lime Juice
2 Tablespoons Curry Powder

6 Skinless, Boneless Organic Chicken Breasts, Cubed
1 Teaspoon Hot Pepper Sauce (Check Ingredients)
2 Clove Garlic, Chopped or Put Through a Press

Combine nut butter, tamari or soy sauce, lime juice, curry powder, garlic and hot pepper sauce. Place the chicken breasts in the marinade and refrigerate. Let the chicken marinate at least 2 hours or overnight. Preheat a grill to high, weave the chicken onto wooden skewers (soak them first to prevent them catching on fire) and grill for approx. 5 min on each side.

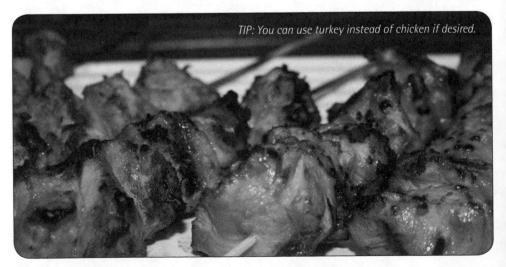

TIP: You can use turkey instead of chicken if desired.

Buffalo Chicken Rolls • Servings: 4

A good alternative to chicken wings which are usually fried in bad oils. This is also much fancier a dish.

4 Boneless Chicken Breasts
5 Tablespoons Blue Cheese, Crumbled
2 Tablespoons Butter, Melted

¼ Cup Hot Pepper Sauce (check ingredients)
Romaine Lettuce
Celery and Celery Leaves

Place chicken breasts between sheet of waxed or parchment paper. Pound the chicken breasts down to a 1/4 inch thickness. In a large glass bowl, make the marinade by mixing together the butter and hot pepper sauce. Add the chicken into the marinade, turning to coat; cover and refrigerate 15 - 30 minutes. Preheat the oven to 400F. Remove the chicken from the marinade and spoon 1 tablespoon of the blue cheese onto the center of each chicken breast. Fold in the sides, rolling the chicken around the blue cheese. Secure with wooden picks.

Place the chicken rolls in a baking pan. Bake in 400F oven for 30 minutes or until chicken is fork tender. Set the temperature control at broil or 450F. Arrange the oven rack so the chicken is about 8 inches from the heat. Broil the chicken for about 5 minutes or until brown. Remove the wooden picks from the chicken. Arrange lettuce and chicken on platter. Garnish with celery and celery leaves and remaining blue cheese.

• •

Easy Cuban Style Sauteed Chicken Breasts • Servings: 4

This is a great simple recipe for chicken to be added atop a salad or with steamed vegetables.

4 Boneless, Skinless Chicken Breasts
4 Cloves of Garlic, Mashed and Chopped
3 Limes, Juiced
1 Teaspoon Sea Salt

1 Tablespoon Balsamic or Apple Cider Vinegar
1 Teaspoon Dried Oregano
2 Tablespoons Olive Oil (or as needed for sauteeing)
2 Tablespoons Grapeseed Oil (or as needed for sauteeing)

Slice the chicken breasts evenly in half. Cover with wax paper and use a mallet to pound them on both sides, until they are approximately 1/4 thin. Place in a glass bowl with the rest of the marinade ingredients, and refrigerate for at least one hour, (Longer will be even better).

When ready to cook, place an equal amount of olive oil and grapeseed oil in a pan, just enough to coat the bottom. Sautée the chicken at low to medium heat on each side until golden and cooked through (about 5 minutes each side, it might need longer if thicker).

• •

Fish Fry Dinner • Servings: 4

With very minor change to the typical fried fishs, you can enjoy fish that your children won't feed to the cat.

1 To 2 Pounds of Wild Caught Fresh or Frozen Fish of Your Choice, such as:
Grouper, Red Snapper, Amberjack, Cod or White Fish of any Variety
1 to 2 Tablespoons Coconut Oil
3 to 4 Tablespoons of Coconut Flour
Optional: Salt, Pepper, Cayenne, Lemon Pepper Lemon Wedges

Heat the coconut oil in a large skillet. (This process takes very little time, but requires your full attention.) Dust or dredge your fish in the coconut flour and lightly season to taste. Sauté the fish in coconut oil over medium high heat for approximately 3 to 4 minutes per side, depending on the thickness of your fish, until the coating is golden brown and the fish is cooked, and flakes to the touch. Garnish with lemon wedges. Serve immediately.

Fancy Salmon • Servings: 4

This is an exclusive restaurant style recipe. It is great for a quiet dinner or for entertaining guests.

1 Tablespoon Olive Oil
2 Shallots, Chopped
¼ Cup Red Wine Vinegar
2 Tablespoons Soy Sauce or Tamari
¼ Cup Fresh Lemon Juice
¼ Teaspoon Cayenne Pepper
1 Tablespoon Fresh Ginger, Chopped
2 Tablespoons Fresh Cilantro, Chopped
4 Wild Caught Salmon Steaks, Skinless

Sauce: Mix first 7 ingredients in a saucepan. Cook until shallots are soft (about 3 minutes). Remove from heat. Mix in cilantro. Baste the salmon on both sides. Grill or broil 10 minutes on each side, turning once and basting frequently with sauce.

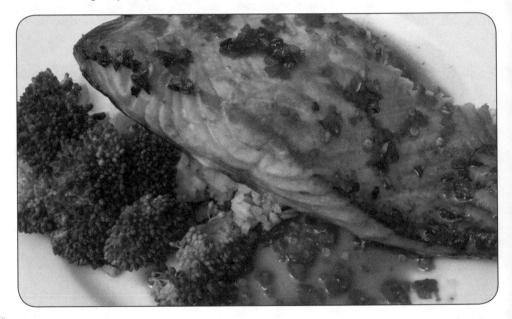

Teriyaki Salmon • Servings: 4

Simple and delicious.

¼ Cup Olive Oil
¼ Cup Fresh Lemon Juice
¼ Cup Soy Sauce or Tamari
1 Teaspoon Mustard

1 Teaspoon Ground Ginger
¼ Teaspoon Garlic Powder
4 Wild Salmon Steaks

TIP: This is a quicker version of the recipe above. It is great for a quick meal and for leftovers.

In a glass pan, combine the first 6 ingredients. Mix well. Set aside 1/4 cup for basting and refrigerate. Place the salmon into a glass dish and let marinate for 1 hour in the refrigerator. Drain and discard marinade. Place the salmon on a broiler pan or grill. Broil or grill for 4-5 minutes. Brush with reserved marinade. Turn and broil or grill for 5 more minutes or as desired.

Crispy Salmon Cakes with Red Pepper and Tomato Sauce

• Servings: 4

These can be saved for a special occasion or made ahead of time and Frozen for a quick meal later.

Salmon Cakes:

1 Can Wild Caught Salmon, Drained
1 Green Onion, Finely Chopped
1 Tablespoon Cilantro, Finely Chopped
1 Tablespoon Red Pepper, Finely Chopped

2 Tablespoons Coconut Oil
⅓ Cup Almond Flour, Plus ¼ Cup for Dredging
1 Teaspoon Fresh Lemon Juice
1 Egg

Sweet Red Pepper and Tomato Sauce

2 Cups Chopped Red Pepper
1 Container Grape Tomatoes
2 Green Onions, Finely Sliced
2 Tablespoons Cilantro, Finely Chopped

1 Teaspoon Sesame Oil
2 Tablespoons Balsamic Vinegar
1 Teaspoon Chili Powder

Salmon Cakes: Makes 4 Cakes: Mix all ingredients together in a bowl until well combined. Form 4 round patties, 2 inches in diameter. Spread remaining almond flour on a piece of waxed paper or plate. Coat patties in almond flour, pressing to form firm, well-coated cakes. Heat oil in a frying pan over medium heat. Pan fry cakes 3-4 minutes on each side or until slightly brown and crisp.

Sweet Red Pepper and Tomato Sauce: Put all ingredients into a blender or food processor and blend to desired consistency. Pour into a saucepan and heat.

Smoked Salmon Tartar • Servings: 2

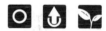

This recipe is so quick and easy to make and will even appeal to those new to raw foods. The key to this dish is to buy very high quality smoked salmon.

4 Ounce Package Sliced Smoked Salmon
1 Tablespoon Shallot, Finely Chopped
1 Tablespoon Olive Oil
1 Tablespoon Fresh Dill
1 Lemon, Thinly Sliced

Chop the smoked salmon into small rough dice. Combine in a bowl with the olive oil, shallots and chopped fresh dill and mix until combined. To serve, use a 1 cup measuring cup (preferably round) as a mold, and pack with the tartar. Turn out onto plate and garnish with a small sprig of dill, the thinly sliced lemon. You can serve with some wasabi cream sauce if desired. To make your own just mix mayonnaise with some prepared wasabi (just check ingredients).

> *Wild Caught Fish – Fish is a very nutritious food, but just like beef, a distinction must be made. Farm raised fish are fed grains instead of their natural diet of krill and shrimp, thus denaturing their natural composition. For example, wild caught salmon is high in the antioxidant astaxanthin, which is depleted once farm raised. Farm raised salmon has also been shown to contain 16 times more PCB's than wild salmon. Wild caught fish is a great source of omega-3s, calcium, selenium, and protein. Fish helps regulate blood sugar, improve heart function, helps the brain and mood, prevents disease, and boosts metabolism. To avoid fish high in mercury contamination, choose smaller fish, from the coldest waters, and furthest away from the Atlantic Ocean.*

Roasted Vegetable Lasagna · Servings: 4-6

This recipe takes a bit of preparation but is well worth it.
Make it when you have some extra time and use the leftovers for lunches.

1 Large Eggplant, Sliced into 1/4 Inch Rounds
1/2 Pound Medium Mushrooms, Cut into 1/4 Inch Slices
3 Small Zucchini, Sliced Lengthwise into 1/4 inch Slices
2 Sweet Red Peppers, Cut into 6 Pieces Each
3 Tablespoons Olive Oil
1 Clove Garlic, Minced
1 (15 Ounce) Container Ricotta Cheese (Drained)
1/2 Teaspoon Pepper
1/4 Cup Parmesan Cheese, Grated
1 Egg
1 Teaspoon Sea Salt
1 (26 ounce) Jar Pasta Sauce (Check Ingredients) or Homemade Sauce
2 Cups Mozzarella Cheese, Grated
3 Tablespoons Basil, Minced

Spread eggplant and mushrooms onto a baking pan. Place zucchini and red pepper on a second pan. Combine the oil and garlic; brush over both sides of vegetables. Sprinkle with salt and pepper. Bake uncovered at 400°F for 15 minutes. Turn vegetables over and cook 15 minutes more. Remove eggplant and mushrooms. Bake zucchini and red pepper 5-10 minutes until edges are browned. In a bowl, combine the ricotta cheese, parmesan cheese, and egg. Spread about 1/2 cup pasta sauce in a 9" x 13" x 2". glass baking dish. Layer with half the ricotta cheese mixture, half of the vegetables, a third of the pasta sauce, and 2/3 cup of the mozzarella cheese. Sprinkle with basil. Repeat layers.

Top with remaining pasta sauce. Cover and bake at 350°F for 40 minutes. Uncover, sprinkle with remaining cheese. Bake 5-10 minutes longer or until edges are bubbly and cheese is melted. Let stand for 10 minutes before cutting.

. . . .

Stuffed Porto Patty · Servings: 4

Portabello mushrooms are a great meat alternative because they are thick, meaty, and very filling.

4 Medium Portabello Mushrooms
1 Large Tomato, Diced
1 Yellow Bell Pepper, Diced
6-8 Kalamata Olives, Sliced
4 Leaves Chopped Fresh Basil
1/2 Small Red Onion, Diced

2 Teaspoons Garlic, Minced
2 Tablespoons Butter,
1/4 Teaspoon Sea Salt (optional)
1/4 Teaspoon Course Black Pepper
Goat Cheese Crumbles

Optional: 2 handfuls fresh spinach.

Melt butter and garlic until tender. Trim stems off mushrooms and wipe off any dirt with damp towel. Brush insides of mushrooms with half of melted butter and garlic. Sautee peppers, onion, tomatoes, basil, spinach (if desired), olives and black pepper for 3-4 minutes with rest of butter and garlic. Meanwhile, grill mushrooms top up for approx. 4 minutes. Turn over and top with veggie mixture and cheese. Continue grilling until cheese is soft.

Oven option: bake mushrooms for 10 minutes, top with remaining ingredients and cook for another 20-30 minutes or until done.

Sides

You will not see a large amount of recipes here because most side dishes consist of simple raw, steamed, or roasted vegetables that do not require a recipe at all. For instance, you can combine any meat with 2-3 vegetables for a healthy, satisfying meal. However, for a change of pace at times, more elaborate recipes may be desired. Here is a small collection of side dishes.

Fried Rice • Servings: 4

This recipe is better than the restaurant version. It is quick and can easily turn into a complete dinner with the addition of chopped chicken or turkey. It is great as leftovers too! You can add extra vegetables or protein- just adjust the ingredients accordingly.

3 Tablespoons Coconut Oil
4 Cups Brown Rice, Cooked
1 1/2 Teaspoon Soy Sauce or Tamari
2 Eggs, Slightly Beaten
1/4 Teaspoon Fresh Ground Pepper

Optional:
1/4 Cup Scallions, Chopped
1/4 Cup Corn
1/4 Cup Peas
1/4 Cup Chopped Carrots

Heat the oil in a large skillet, and add the rice, soy sauce or tamari, pepper and optional ingredients. Cook over medium-high heat, stirring often, for about 6 minutes. Add the eggs and stir briskly so they cook and break into small bits throughout the rice. As soon as the egg is set, remove and serve.

· ·

Zesty Lemon Quinoa • Servings: 4

Although quinoa is great on it's own, the extra spice of this dish makes it very unique.

1 Cup Quinoa
1/2 Cup Toasted Pine Nuts or Toasted Pecans
1/4 Cup Olive Oil
1/4 Cup Lemon Juice
2 Teaspoon Freshly Grated Lemon Zest
1 Teaspoon Ground Cumin
1/4 Teaspoon Cayenne
1/2 Cup Chopped Flat-Leaf Parsley
Sea Salt and Fresh ground black pepper

Rinse quinoa in a fine strainer for a few seconds. Transfer to a medium saucepan, add 1 teaspoon sea salt and 1 1/4 cups water. Bring to a boil, cover, and reduce to a simmer. Cook until water is completely absorbed, about 18 to 20 minutes. Transfer quinoa to a medium bowl along with pine nuts, lemon zest, cumin, cayenne, parsley, drizzle with lemon juice and olive oil. Season with salt and pepper; toss until well combined. Serve warm or at room temperature.

· ·

Garlic-Roasted Cauliflower • Servings: 4

The roasted garlic compliments the cauliflower perfectly.

1 Head Cauliflower, Separated and Roasted in Florets
1 or 2 Cloves Minced Garlic, Extremely Lightly Sautéed in Olive Oil
1 Small Jar Capers

While cauliflower is roasting, lightly sauté the minced garlic in the olive oil. Add capers, juice and all, to the oil and lightly heat through. Pour this sauce over the cauliflower once it is roasted and serve immediately.

Tip: You don't want the olive oil to become too hot – just let the flavor of the olive oil infuse the oil.

Boosted Broccoli • Servings: 4

Broccoli is a super vegetable on its own full of vitamins and nutrients but when combined with the healthy omega 3's of anchovies- it is amazingly nutritious. When heated, the anchovies just melt into the sauce. People who don't like anchovies will eat this dish.

4 Anchovy Fillets
2 Tablespoons Olive Oil
1 Head Broccoli Cut into Florets
3 Cloves Garlic, Sliced Thinly
1 Lemon, Juiced

TIP: The crunchy garlic slices in this dish are also a great topping for salads.

Place the anchovy fillets in a small, cold skillet and slowly heat over low heat (do not overheat). You can use a fork to break up the anchovies as they heat. Once melted, turn off the heat.
In a separate pan, heat olive oil on medium heat (do not let it smoke) and add the garlic. Stir until light brown. Use a fork to take the garlic slices out of the pan and drain them on paper towels.
Transfer the melted anchovies to a small bowl and add 1 tablespoon of the garlic oil and the lemon juice. Stir until mixed. Steam the broccoli over boiling water until just tender- no more than 5 minutes. Put broccoli in a serving dish with the fried garlic slices and the anchovy sauce.

Broccoli – Broccoli is a super-vegetable. Among many other things, it is high in isothiocanates (anticancer phytochemicals). Broccoli is incredible for women because of its high levels of indoles, an antioxidant which has a positive effect on estrogen. It is high in sulforaphone which helps fight carcinogens in the body. Broccoli is high in protein, fiber, potassium, calcium, and vitamin C. Its vitamin C content can rival citrus. Its calcium content can rival milk and is more usable in the body!

Mashed NO-tatoes • Servings: 4

This is a good alternative to high carbohydrate mashed potatoes.
This is not only low carb but it is highly nutritious. Use it in place of potatoes or rice.

1 Head Cauliflower
Sea Salt and Black Pepper to Taste
2 Tablespoons Organic Butter
1-2 Cloves of Garlic, Optional

Steam cauliflower until very soft (you can also boil it but this is not recommended as a lot of the nutrients are lost). Chop up cauliflower and put in a food processor or blender with butter, salt, pepper, and garlic if desired. Blend to desired consistency.

• •

Smashed Sweet Potatoes • Servings: 4

Kids will love this. Add ingredients according to your personal taste.

3-4 Large Sweet Potatoes
1 Granny Smith Apple
1-2 Tablespoons Butter or Coconut Oil

Cinnamon
Stevia
Sea Salt

Peel and cut up sweet potatoes into chunks. Boil until tender. Meanwhile, melt butter or coconut oil (1-2 tablespoons) in a skillet and cut up apple. Saute apple in butter until soft. Add cinnamon, stevia, and salt to taste. Add apple mixture to sweet potatoes and mash with a potato masher or electric mixer.

Zucchini Boats • Servings: 4

Impress your friends with this delicious and beautifully presented dish.
You will want to double this recipe!

2 Medium Zucchini
¾ Pound Ground Turkey
1 Small Onion, Chopped
1 Cup Raw Cheese (or Cheese Alternative), Shredded (Optional)
2 Tablespoons Fruit Sweetened Ketchup or Tomato Paste

½ Teaspoon Sea Salt
¼ Teaspoon Pepper
½ Cup Sliced Fresh Mushrooms
½ Cup Sweet Red Peppers
½ Cup Chopped Green Peppers

Trim the ends of the zucchini. Cut in half lengthwise. Scoop out pulp, laving a ½ inch shell. Finely chop pulp. In a skillet, cook ground turkey, zucchini pulp, onion, mushrooms, and peppers until meat is brown, drain. Remove from heat. Add ½ cup cheese, ketchup, sea salt, and pepper. Mix well. Spoon into the zucchini shells Place in a buttered 13 x 9 x 2 inch baking dish. Sprinkle with remaining cheese if desired. Bake uncovered at 350°F for 30 minutes.

• •

Sunflower Herb Pate • Servings: 1-2

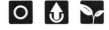

Great as a snack or lunchtime accompaniment

1 Cup Soaked Raw Sunflower Seeds
2 Tablespoons of Water
1 Tablespoon Lemon Juice
½ Teaspoon Crushed Garlic (1 Clove)

¼ Teaspoon Sea Salt
Dash Cayenne or Black Pepper
1 Tablespoon Minced Green or Red Onion
2 Teaspoons. Minced Fresh Dill Weed, Basil, Cilantro, or Parsley

Place the sunflower seeds, water, lemon juice, garlic, salt and cayenne pepper in food processor and mix into paste. Stop occasionally to scrape down the sides with a spatula. Transfer into a small bowl and mix in red onion and dill weed. Store in well sealed container and refrigerate for up to 5 days.

Variations: Add 1/3 cup of sundried tomatoes to the food processor. Replace sunflower seeds with raw pumpkins seeds.

• •

Quick Sauerkraut • Servings: 6 Cups

Most sauerkraut recipes require days of tending. While this raw method is preferred,
most people don't have the time or space to do it. This cooked version speeds up the process. Cabbage is natures broom as it helps clear out your intestines and has a ton of nutrients.

1 Head Green Cabbage, Outer Leaves Removed, Thinly Sliced
½ Cup Distilled White Vinegar
1 Tablespoon Coarse Sea Salt

In a medium saucepan, combine cabbage, vinegar, salt, and 1¼ cups water. Cover, and cook over medium heat, stirring occasionally until cabbage is tender (30-35 minutes) Add more water if necessary. Store in the refrigerator for up to 2 weeks.

> *Avocados – Avocados are a great fat that is often overlooked. Like olive oil, it is high in monounsaturated fats like oleic acid. Its mono and beta sitosterols have been shown to help lower cholesterol and prevent heart disease. Avocados contain the antioxidant lutein, which supports healthy skin and eyes. Avocados are high in fiber, folate, vitamin A, and beta carotene. They are a filling snack or a great addition to many different foods.*

Green Bean Almondine • Servings: 4

Most green bean recipes call for the beans to be cooked so long that much of the nutrients are lost. In this recipe they remain completely intact.

3 Tablespoons Lemon Juice
8 Tablespoons Olive Oil
1 Clove of Garlic, Minced
1 Tablespoons Onion Minced
½ Teaspoon Dry Mustard

½ Teaspoon Sea Salt
¼ Fresh Ground Pepper
4 Cups Greens Beans, French Cut
2 Cups Mushrooms, Wiped and Sliced
1 Cup Almonds. Sliced

TIP: Use the slicer blade in a food processor to French cut the beans. Just put a whole handful in at a time and press down.

Combine ingredients for marinade and pour over beans, mushrooms and almonds. Toss well. Allow to marinate for 2 hours in a dehydrator or overnight in the refrigerator. Serve chilled or just slightly warmed.

• •

Curry Eggs • Servings: 6

This is a great meatless dish that is high in protein and very satisfying.
It takes a shortcut by using store bought organic marinara sauce but you can also make your own.

2 Tablespoons Coconut Oil
1 Onion, Thinly Sliced
3 Cups (24 ounces) Organic Crushed Tomatoes or Homemade Marinara Sauce
1 Tablespoon Curry Powder
4 Cloves Garlic, Minced
2 Tablespoons Fresh Ginger, Peeled and Minced or Microplaned
8 Hard Boiled Eggs
Salt And Pepper to Taste

TIP: If you are not following the advanced plan, this can be served over brown rice or quinoa.

Heat oil in a large skillet over meduim-high heat. Add onion, garlic, and ginger. Season with salt and pepper to taste; cook, stirring occasionally until onion begins to soften (4-5 minutes). Add curry powder and cook while stirring about 30 seconds. Add marinara sauce and eggs; cook just to heat through (2-3 minutes), stirring gently to avoid breaking up eggs.

• •

Greek Greens • Servings: 4

Greens are great on their own sautéed in some olive or coconut oil, but
for a more ethnic flair, this is a great variation

1 Tablespoon Coconut Oil
½ Red or Yellow Onion, Sliced into Rings
2 Pounds Spinach, Swiss Chard, Kale, or Collards, (Ribs Removed)
½ Teaspoon Grated Lemon Peel
¼ Cup Black or Kalamata Olives, Pitted and Sliced.
Juice of One Lemon
¼ Teaspoon Sea Salt
¼ Teaspoon Pepper
¼ Cup Crumbled Feta Cheese

Heat the oil in a very large skillet that will fit all of the greens. Sautée the onion until softens. Add greens and sautée for 2-3 minutes. Add lemon juice, lemon peel, salt, pepper, and olives and cook for a few minutes more to combine. Add crumbled feta and stir. Serve immediately.

Sauces/ Dips

Use traditional hard-to-damage fats and oils in cooking and baking. This includes butter and/or ghee (organic from grass-fed cows), extra virgin olive oil, expeller-pressed nut oils (walnut, sesame), and coconut oil.

Pesto Sauce

This is great on eggs, baked with cauliflower with steamed vegetables, over whole wheat pasta or spiral sliced zucchini, as a dip...use your imagination.

3 Cups Chopped Fresh Basil
1 Cup Extra Virgin Olive Oil
2 Tablespoons Garlic, Minced
$\frac{1}{2}$ Cup Pine Nuts or Walnuts Ground Fine
$\frac{2}{3}$ Cup Grated Parmesan
$\frac{1}{2}$ Teaspoon Chili Powder, Optional

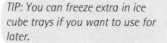
TIP: You can freeze extra in ice cube trays if you want to use for later.

Place the basil in a blender. Pour in about 1 tablespoon of the olive oil, and blend the basil into a paste. Gradually add pine nuts or walnuts, cheese, garlic, chili powder if desired, and drizzle in remaining oil. Continue to blend until smooth.

Worcestershire Sauce

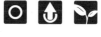

Most store bought Worcestershire sauces contain sugar so here is a homemade version that you can store in your refrigerator.

$\frac{1}{2}$ Cup Apple Cider Vinegar
2 Tablespoons Soy Sauce or Tamari

2 Tablespoons Water
Stevia or Xylitol to Taste
$\frac{1}{4}$ Teaspoon Ground Ginger
1-2 Anchovy Fillets, Chopped

$\frac{1}{4}$ Teaspoon Dry Mustard
$\frac{1}{4}$ Teaspoon Onion Powder
$\frac{1}{4}$ Teaspoon Garlic Powder
$\frac{1}{8}$ Teaspoon Cinnamon
$\frac{1}{8}$ Teaspoon Pepper
1 Jalepeño, Chopped (Optional)

Place all ingredients in a medium saucepan and stir thoroughly. Bring to a boil, stirring constantly. Simmer 1 minute. Cool. Store in the refrigerator.

15 Minute Pasta Sauce • Servings: 2

Everyone needs a simple tomato based sauce in their recipe list.

2 Tablespoons Olive Oil
4 Pinch Pepper, Fresh Ground
$\frac{1}{2}$ Cup Onion, Finely Chopped
2 Garlic Cloves, Minced
1 Can Tomatoes (28 Ounces), Crushed

Place a large heavy pan over moderate heat. Add the oil, garlic, pepper and onion. Cook for 5 minutes, or until fragrant. Add crushed tomatoes. Reduce heat and simmer, stirring occasionally for 10 minutes. Season with salt and your favorite chopped fresh herb (basil, fresh oregano, or fresh coriander). Fresh herbs make a big difference in quality and flavor. Serve over pasta.

TIP: You can make a large batch and freeze sauce in portion sizes in containers. If you freeze the sauce right after you make it, you will capture the flavor.

Puttanesca Sauce • Servings: 4

This is a simple sauce that can be made with items you have on hand.

¼ Cup Olive Oil
1 Can Plum Tomatoes (28 Ounces), Drained
1 Large Garlic Cloves, Peeled
6 Anchovy Fillets, Drained
½ Cup Parsley, Finely Chopped

3 Teaspoon Capers
⅛ Teaspoon Red Pepper Flakes, Crushed
20 Black Kalamata Olives, Pitted
1 Small Bunch Fresh Basil Leaves
Grated Parmesan

Heat the olive oil over low heat in a large skillet. Add the garlic and mashed anchovies, stir until almost dissolved, about 5 minutes. Stir in the capers, red pepper and olives; cook 1 minute. Add the basil and tomatoes; bring to a slow boil. Reduce the heat and simmer 10- 12 minutes. Add a little of the reserved juice if the sauce seems too dry. Remove from the heat and stir in the parsley. Pour the sauce over the cooked pasta. Serve parmesan on the side.

TIP: This sauce can be served over whole wheat pasta, spiral sliced zucchini, or spaghetti squash.

Taco Seasoning Mix • Servings: Enough for 1 Pound of Meat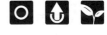

Making your own seasonings is very easy and so much healthier than the kind you buy in a package. Why Most store bought seasonings are loaded with salt, artificial ingredients, and dangerous additives!

2 Tablespoon Chili Powder
2 Tablespoon Flour, Optional
½ Teaspoon Salt
2 Teaspoon Cumin

½ Teaspoon Onion Powder
½ Teaspoon Garlic Powder
2 Teaspoon Oregano
½ Teaspoon Cayenne Pepper

Combine all ingredients in a zip lock bag and shake until completely mixed. Add to browned ground beef along with ½-¾ cup water and cook until reduced to desired consistency.

TIP: When making taco filling, add 1/2 cup salsa to the pan while heating.

Mayonnaise • Servings: 1½ cups

This is a great way to make your own mayonnaise without a lot of fuss.

2 Egg Yolks
1 Tablespoon Apple Cider Vinegar
1 Teaspoon Dry Mustard
½ Teaspoon Salt
1¼ Cups Olive Oil

TIP: You can also mix in a bowl with a whisk, adding the oil drop by drop at first and then graduating into a thin stream.

In a food processor, combine egg yolks, apple cider vinegar, dry mustard, and salt. With machine running very slowly add olive oil through the feed tube.

30 Minutes Most Maximized Living meals are designed to be ready within 30 minutes. This takes less time than it does driving to a restaurant, deciding on a meal, and eating. Most importantly, it is much healthier.

Balsamic Mustard Sauce • Servings: About 4

This sauce is versatile and delicious. It can be used on chicken, turkey, steak or salmon.

1 Tablespoon Olive Oil
Kosher Salt and Ground Pepper
¹/₂ Cup Balsamic Vinegar
¹/₄ Cup Dijon Mustard (No Sugar – Check the Label)

Heat oil in a large skillet over medium heat. Add vinegar to skillet; boil until syrupy, 1 to 2 miutes. Remove from heat; whisk in mustard and any accumulated juices from the cooked meat. Serve sauce with 4 grass-fed beef strip steaks (each 6 to 8 ounces and about ³/₄ inch thick) or 4-6 grilled or sautéed chicken breasts or thighs.

. . . .

Tzatziki Dip (Yogurt Dip) • Servings: About 4

This traditional Greek recipe is usually made with cucumbers. In this version, we replace the cucumbers with Swiss Chard for a different twist on this classic.

1 Cup Swiss Chard Leaves, Finely Chopped (Ribs Removed)
1 Clove Garlic
¹/₄ Teaspoon Sea Salt
1 Cup Plain Yogurt
1 Tablespoon Extra Virgin Olive Oil
1 Tablespoon Lemon Juice, Freshly Squeezed
Dash of Cayenne Pepper

Bring a 1-2 quart saucepan, half filled with water, to a boil. Add the chopped swiss chard leaves and cook until tender, about 2-5 minutes. While the chard is cooking, prepare a bowl with water and ice for an ice bath. When the chard is cooked, strain with a fine mesh strainer and put into the ice bath to stop the cooking. Drain and set aside. Using a mortar and pestle, grind the garlic and salt into a paste. In a medium sized bowl, stir in the yogurt, chard, garlic, olive oil, lemon juice, and cayenne pepper. Set aside. Serve with raw vegetables.

. . . .

Hummus • Servings: 4-6

This is delicious and good with grainless crackers, veggies, in a veggie sandwich, etc.

1 Can Chick Peas
2 Cloves Garlic
3 Tablespoons Extra Virgin Olive Oil
Lemon Juice (adjust amount to desired consistency or taste)
Sea Salt

Optional: Tahini (sesame paste)
Fresh Parsley
Paprika
Cumin
Cayenne

Put chick peas, garlic, and olive oil into food processor.
All other ingredients are added to suit taste and consistency.

Saturated fats are needed by your body's cell membranes to transfer toxins OUT and nutrients IN. Great saturated fat comes from grass-fed meat, coconut, avocados, and nuts.

Baba Ganoush (Eggplant Dip) • Servings: 4-6

This traditional middle eastern dish is very impressive in taste and presentation without a lot of fuss.

2 Globe Eggplants (about 2 pounds)
3 Tablespoons Extra Virgin Olive Oil
2 Tablespoons Tahini (Sesame Paste)
1 Clove Garlic, Finely Minced or Pressed
1/2 Teaspoon Ground Cumin

2 1/2 Tablespoons Lemon Juice, Freshly Squeeze
3/4 Teaspoon Sea Salt
Cayenne Pepper
1 Tablespoon Cilantro, Chopped

Preheat the oven to 375ºF. Cut the eggplant in half lengthwise and brush with olive oil. Place on a baking sheet, cut side down and roast until very tender, about 35 minutes. Place the eggplant in a colander to drain and cool for 15 minutes, then scoop the flesh out of the skin. Combine the eggplant, remaining olive oil, tahini, garlic, cumin, 2 tablespoons of the lemon juice, the salt, and a pinch of cayenne in the workbowl of a food processor. Pulse until the eggplant is smooth but retains some of its texture.

Allow the baba ganoush to sit for one hour at room temperature, then season it to taste with additional lemon juice, salt, and cayenne. Toss in cilantro and serve with raw vegetables.

• •

Easy Guacamole • Servings: 1-2

This is SO easy and healthy. If you are in a rush, use only the first three ingredients.
You can alter it to your liking with additional spices.

1 Avocado, Mashed
2-3 Teaspoons Salsa
Sea Salt to Taste

Optional: Chili Powder
Onion Powder
Garlic, Chopped or Pressed

Cut avocado in half, remove pit, and use a spoon to scoop out the middle. Smash avocado with a fork, add salsa, and stir. Enjoy immediately. If you make ahead add some lemon juice to keep it from browning.

> *TIP: To cut an avocado, first cut all the way around it lengthwise with a knife and separate. Lightly tap the knife into the pit inside and twist. The pit will pop right out. You can then use a spoon to scoop the avocado out or slice it right in the skin and then turn inside out to remove.*

• •

White Bean Dip • Servings:1½ Cups

1 Can Cannelloni Beans
(or Other White Beans) Rinsed and Drained
1/4 Cup Olive Oil
2 Tablespoons Lemon Juice
1 Teaspoon Fresh Rosemary
1 Clove Garlic, Minced
Sea Salt to Taste
Fresh Ground Pepper to Taste

Puree all ingredients in food processor until smooth. Garnish with fresh rosemary sprigs. Drizzle with olive oil if desired.

Bagna Cauda (Italian Anchovy Dip) • Servings: About 4

This is absolutely amazing. Even people who don't like fish will love this recipe. It is a great way to get in the good fats as it is loaded with healthy Omega 3's!

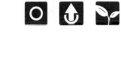

¹/₃ Cups Extra Virgin Olive Oil
2 Tablespoons Butter
6 Anchovy Fillets
6 Sardines (Skinless Works Best)
or 12 Anchovy Fillets (No Sardines)
3 Cloves Garlic Pressed or Chopped
Assorted Fresh Vegetables

Put all ingredients except vegetables into a blender and blend for a few seconds. Transfer to a saucepan and heat on low for about 15 minutes (DO NOT HEAT OLIVE OIL TOO HIGH). Season with sea salt and pepper. Serve with an assortment of raw vegetables like: lettuce leaves, celery, red bell peppers, broccoli, cauliflower, carrots, zucchini, cabbage etc. You can even put this in a fondue pot or crockpot for entertaining.

· ·

Olivata Dip or Spread • Servings: 1 cup

This rich olive paste is great for whole wheat bread, grainless crackers, or as a spread on a sandwich.

1 Tablespoon Water
1 Tablespoon Balsamic Vinegar
1 Tablespoon Red Wine Vinegar
¹/₄ Cup Sun Dried Tomatoes
¹/₂ Cup Pitted Kalamata Olives

1 Tablespoon Chopped Fresh Basil
1 Tablespoon Olive Oil
¹/₂ Teaspoon Chopped Garlic
¹/₄ Teaspoon Pepper
¹/₈ Teaspoon Salt

Combine first 4 ingredients in a small saucepan. Bring to a boil over medium-high heat; reduce heat, and simmer, stirring occasionally, 1 to 2 minutes or until liquid is absorbed and tomatoes have plumped. Process tomato mixture with the remaining ingredients in a food processor or blender until smooth, scraping down the sides if necessary.

> *Without fat, your body cannot absorb and utilize the vitamins and minerals found in food.*

· ·

Herbed Butters • Servings: 4

These butters kick up the flavor and make for a beautiful accompaninment to your meal. Try different flavor combinations.

4 Tablespoons Unsalted Butter
1 Tablespoon Fresh Herbs or ¹/₂ Tablespoon Dried Herbs
Mixture of Herbs: (your choice) Parsley, Sage, Chives,
Basil, Thyme, Tarragon, Rosemary, Garlic, Sun Dried Tomatoes.
Salt, Pepper

Let butter soften and then blend together with selected herbs and spices.

> *TIP: You can keep it in a sealable container in the refrigerator or freezer or form it into a log, wrap in waxed paper, and chill. When cold, you can slice it into beautiful herbed butter medallions.*

Dressings

Salad dressings, while they seem harmless because they are added to a heap of vegetables, are perfect hiding spots for harmful ingredients. Most commercial salad dressings contain some form of bad fats, sugars, additives and preservatives, and excessive table salt. If you are eating out, ask for olive oil and vinegar or bring your own. At home, you can try these healthy dressings.

Roasted Shallot Salad Dressing • Servings: About 4

The family-favorite salad dressing!

1 Small Bag of Shallots
Coconut Oil

Balsamic Vinegar
Extra Virgin Olive Oil

Peel and slice the shallots; then sauté them in a tiny bit of coconut oil until they begin to caramelize. Deglaze the pan with some balsamic vinegar, and remove from heat. Pour the shallots and vinegar into a blender, and add more balsamic vinegar – approximately one cup. Turn the blender on, at first to a low setting, and then increasing the speed as the shallots are incorporated. Once the high setting has been established, stream in approximately two cups of extra virgin olive oil, very slowly so that the dressing will emulsify. (Amounts listed can be varied to your liking.)

• •

Caesar Dressing • Servings: About 4

This is a classic dressing usually paired with only chopped romaine lettuce. Simple and delicious.

1 Egg
$1/2$ Cup White Wine Vinegar
2 Tablespoons Lemon Juice
2 Cloves Garlic, Minced
$1/2$ Teaspoon Sea Salt

$1/4$ Teaspoon Pepper
$3/4$ Cup Olive Oil
$1/3$ Cup Freshly Grated Raw Parmesan Cheese
1-2 Sardine Fillets, Optional

In a blender add all ingredients except olive oil. Blend well. While the processor is running, slowly add the olive oil. Use immediately or refrigerate up to one week.

• •

Greek Dressing • Servings: About 4

This dressing is great on any salad or over raw or freshly steamed vegetables. Traditional Greek salads consist of mixed greens, tomatoes, cucumber, sliced red onions, olives, and feta cheese.

4 Tablespoons Extra Virgin Olive Oil
2 Tablespoons Fresh Lemon Juice
2 Tablespoons Water
1 Tablespoon Feta
1 Tablespoon Chopped Red Onion
1 Teaspoon Sea Salt
$1/2$ Teaspoon Dijon Mustard (No Sugar – Check Label)
3 Large Fresh Basil Leaves

TIP: Feta cheese from sheep or goat's milk is preferable.
TIP: Keeps for about 3 days in an air-tight jar in the refrigerator.

Blend all ingredients until smooth.

Coconut – Coconut products are not only delicious but extremely healthy. Coconut products are high in GOOD fat. 92% of coconut fats are MCFA's (medium chain fatty acids) which metabolize very easily and provide immediate energy. MCFA's are proven in cancer prevention, weight loss, and boosting athletic performance. instead of being stored in the body. Coconuts have antimicrobial, antibacterial, and antiviral properties. They are high in antioxidants, fiber, potassium, magnesium, and low in sugar. Coconut carries vitamins and regulates hormones. Coconut oil is the absolute best to cook with because it can withstand medium to high heat making is less vulnerable to oxidation and rancidity.

Ranch Dressing • Servings: 4-6

Ranch dressing is very popular but typically contains sugars, bad fats, and additives and preservatives. This homemade recipe will appease ranch lovers with none of the negatives.

1 Cup Mayonnaise (see recipe)
1/2 Cup Sour Cream
1/2 Teaspoon Dried Chives
1/2 Teaspoon Dried Parsley
1/2 Teaspoon Dried Dill Weed
1/4 Teaspoon Garlic Powder
1/4 Teaspoon Onion Powder
1/8 Teaspoon Salt
1/8 Teaspoon Ground Black Pepper

In a large bowl, whisk together the mayonnaise, sour cream, chives, parsley, dill, garlic powder, onion powder, salt and pepper. Cover and refrigerate for 30 minutes before serving.

• •

Tomato Basil Dressing • Servings: About 4

For a change of pace, this red dressing is perfect at the start of a meal.

1 Medium Tomato, Roughly Chopped
2 To 4 Tablespoons Apple Cider Vinegar
1/2 Cup Extra Virgin Olive Oil
1/4 Cup Basil Leaves
1/2 Clove Garlic
Salt and Pepper to Taste

Combine all ingredients in a food processor and blend until smooth.

• •

Italian Vinaigrette • Servings: About 4

Nothing beats a great Italian dressing. You can make this one right before you sit down to eat without a lot of fuss.

1/4 Cup Red Wine Vinegar
1 Teaspoon Grated Onion
2 Garlic Cloves, Minced
1 Teaspoon Dijon Mustard
1 Tablespoons Chopped Fresh Oregano or 1 Teaspoons Dried Oregano
3/4 Cup Extra-Virgin Olive Oil
Sea Salt and Freshly Ground Black Pepper to Taste

Combine the vinegar, garlic, mustard, and oregano in a small bowl. Add the olive oil in a slow, steady stream while whisking constantly until all the oil is incorporated. Season with salt and pepper to taste.

> *TIP: You can adjust the flavors of any dressing according to your taste. Just experiment with the quantities and/or substitute spices.*
>
> *TIP: Refrigerate in an airtight container until ready to use or up to 1 week.*

Desserts

Pumpkin Pie • Servings: 8 Slices

Thanksgiving and Christmas are back but without all the sugar!

1 (15 Ounces.) Can Pumpkin Puree (No Sugar- Check the Label)
³/₄ Cup Stevia (Spoonable) or ²/₃ Cup Xylitol
¹/₂ Teaspoon Sea Salt
1 Teaspoon Cinnamon
¹/₂ Teaspoon Ground Ginger
¹/₄ Teaspoon Ground Cloves
4 Ounces Organic Cream
8 Ounces Unsweetened Almond Milk, Original or Vanilla Flavor
1 Almond Pie Crust (see recipe)

Preheat oven to 425°F. Combine all the ingredients. Pour into a cooled almond pie crust. Bake 15 minutes at 425°F. Reduce heat to 350°F and bake for an additional 45 minutes. Cool and garnish with whipped (organic) cream, flavored with cinnamon and stevia.

• •

Almond Pie Crust • Servings: 1 Crust

1¹/₂ Cups Almond Meal or Almond Flour
3 Tablespoons Stevia or Xylitol
3 Tablespoons Melted Butter

Heat oven to 350°F. Melt the butter. Mix the melted butter with the almond meal and stevia. Pat into a glass pie plate with your fingertips. Gently heat in the oven for about 8 minutes. Do not let the crust go brown. Remove from oven and cool.

• •

Chocolate Bark • Servings: 4

Any chocolate lover will approve of this recipe. It makes a great gift as well.

4 Squares Unsweetened Baking Chocolate
1 Tablespoon Butter (optional)
1 Teaspoon Cinnamon (optional)
Stevia and/or Xylitol to taste
1 Handful of Raw Almonds, Raw Pecans, Raw Hazelnuts, or a Combination of Any Raw Nut You Have on Hand.

Melt chocolate and (optional) butter over a double boiler. Add stevia/Xylitol to taste. On a piece of parchment paper in a ¹/₂ sheet pan or on a rimmed cookie sheet, distribute the nuts over the surface. Pour the melted chocolate mixture over the nuts. Cool in refrigerator or freezer. When the bark has hardened, remove from the parchment paper, break into pieces, and store in a plastic bag in the refrigerator or freezer.

> *Nuts and seeds - Cooking or roasting nuts alters the fat and protein to forms that the human body does not recognize. Raw nuts are very healthy but are dense in calories and digest slowly, so exercise caution (eat no more than a handful at a time), particularly if you are trying to lose weight. As an alternative to nuts, go for raw seeds instead.*

Frozen Yogurt • Servings: 4

You don't have to give up delicious treats and desserts.
You are just eating healthier versions of them.

4 Cups Organic Full Fat Yogurt
Stevia to Taste
Optional Add Ins:
Fresh Whole or Pureed Berries
Coconut Milk
Shredded Coconut
Raw Nuts, Chopped
Unsweetened Cocoa Powder
Cocoa Nibs

Mix the ingredients in an ice-cream maker until the desired consistency is reached.

Chocolate Coconut Pudding • Servings: 2

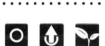

This will be sure to be a favorite go-to treat.
So simple to make and so delicious!

1 can Coconut Milk
Stevia to taste
Unsweetened cocoa to taste

Combine all ingredients and chill in the refrigerator.

TIP: For best results, combine using a blender.

Chocolate Mousse • Servings: 3-4

You won't believe how rich, smooth, and delicious this recipe is.
The surprise ingredient: avocados!

$^1/_2$ Cup Medjool Dates, Soaked
Stevia to Taste
1 Teaspoon Vanilla Extract, Optional
1-$^1/_2$ Cups Mashed Avocado (3 Avocados)
$^3/_4$ Cup Organic Cocoa
$^1/_2$ Cup Water

Place the dates, stevia, and vanilla extract, if using, in a food processor and process until smooth. Add the mashed avocado and cocoa powder and process until creamy. You may need to stop and scrape down the sides of the bowl with a spatula a few times. Add the water and process until smooth. Serve at room temperature or chilled. Stored in a sealed container in the refrigerator. Chocolate Mousse will keep up to 3 days in the refrigerator and 2 weeks in the freezer. Fudgesicles: Freeze the Chocolate Mousse in ice cube trays. Thaw for 5 minutes before serving. Chocolate Sauce or Fondue: Increase the water to 1 cup.

TIP: Delicious alone or served as a fondue with fresh strawberries, bananas, or tangerines.

Zucchini Cake · Servings: 8 Wedges

Zucchini is so versatile because it is great in both savory and sweet dishes.
This cake is moist and delicious.

2 Cups Almond Flour
1 Tablespoon Baking Powder
1/2 Teaspoon Salt
1/2 Teaspoon Stevia
1/4 Cup Walnuts, Chopped
2 Eggs

1/4 Cup Olive Oil
2 Cups Zucchini, Grated
1/2 Cup Half and Half
1 Cup Plain Yogurt
1 Tablespoon Pumpkin Spice

Cream all moist ingredients together except eggs. Add stevia and mix well. Add eggs and mix well. Then add in remaining ingredients and stir. Place in a greased cake pan and bake at 350ºF for 35-40 minutes.

• •

Brownies · Servings: 8 Squares

Use this recipe when you have to bring food for a children's celebration, to share with co-workers, or keep all to yourself.

4 Tablespoons Butter
4 Tablespoons Unsweetened Cocoa Powder
1 1/2 Cup Whey Protein Powder (Chocolate or Vanilla)
2 Teaspoons spoonable Stevia or to Taste
1 Teaspoon Pure Vanilla Extract
1/3 Cup Milled Flaxseed + 2/3 Cup Boiling Water to Gel
1/2 Teaspoon Aluminum Free Baking Powder
1/2 Teaspoon Baking Soda
1/2 Cup Chopped Walnuts, Optional
3/4 Teaspoon Salt
1 Egg

Preheat oven to 275ºF. Melt butter and cocoa powder in a small saucepan on low heat. Stir until smooth. Add protein powder, stevia, salt, vanilla and egg and beat well. Combine milled flaxseed gel, walnuts, baking soda, and baking powder. Add to the chocolate mixture. Mix all ingredients well. Pour mixture into a square baking dish or into 5 ramekins and bake for 10 minutes or into a baking dish and bake for approximately 20 minutes or until a knife or toothpick comes out clean. When done, remove and cool brownies on a wire rack. Serve when cool.

• •

Raw Brownie Balls · Servings: Approximately 10

A great treat for people trying to cut out carbs and sugars because it is very sweet and satisfying!!! It is a kid friendly favorite

1 Cup Walnuts or Pecans
6-10 Pitted Dates, Soaked in Water
1/2 Teaspoon Stevia (or more to taste)
1 Cup Unsweetened Cocoa Powder
2 Teaspoons Ghee or Coconut Oil
1/8 - 1/4 Cup Shredded Coconut, Unsweetened

Put everything in the blender and mix. Shape into one inch balls and refrigerate.

Simple Berry Dessert • Servings: 1

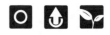

This is a quick recipe that is the perfect snack or light dessert.

2-3 Tablespoons Almond Butter
3-5 Strawberries, Sliced
Coconut Milk
Optional: Blueberries, Blackberries, Raspberries
Stevia
Whey Protein Powder

Place almond butter in a cereal bowl. Add sliced strawberries. Pour coconut milk on top until the mix is thoroughly covered. Best enjoyed immediately. You can sprinkle with protein powder, or stevia and mix until dissolved.

• •

Flan • Servings: 4

This traditional Latin dessert, made without sugar, is a guilt-free option for an after dinner treat.

¼ Cup Xylitol
2 Cups Milk
Pinch of Salt
2 Sticks of Cinnamon

1 Large Egg + 6 Large Egg Yolks
1 Teaspoon Vanilla Extract
Mixed Berries of Your Choice

In a heavy sauce pan, over low heat, simmer milk, salt, xylitol, and cinnamon until the Xylitol dissolves. Remove from the heat and allow to cool to room temperature. In a bowl, mix the egg plus egg yolks, add the vanilla, and mix into the cooled milk mixture. Preheat the oven to 325 Pour the mixture either into individual ramekins or into a 2 quart ovenproof mold. Place this into a larger pan, and set inside a larger pan.

Set in the oven, and carefully fill the larger pan with water, reaching 2/3 of the way up the custard pan. Be careful if you get water in the custard, it will not be creamy. Bake for 1 hour if smaller pans, 1½ hours if large single pan, or until a knife inserted in the center comes out clean. Shake the pan, if it is too wobbly, the custard is not set. Remove from the oven and the water pan, allow to cool to room temperature, and then place in the refrigerator for at least 2 hours before serving. Garnish the top with berries and serve.

> TIP: Unlike a traditional flan, this one has no caramel topping, therefore cannot be flipped over.

• •

Strawberry Sauce • Servings: Any

This sauce can be used in a thousand ways. You can also switch up the berries to make Blueberry Sauce.

Frozen strawberries
Water
Stevia (optional) to taste

Add Frozen strawberries to a sauce pan with a tiny bit of water. Heat the strawberries and water until you begin to get to a syrupy consistency. Taste. Add stevia if desired Finally, add a few more Frozen strawberries to the hot sauce to refresh the color and consistency of the sauce. Continue heating the sauce just until the newly added berries are heated through.

Amazing Almond Cookies • Servings: 10-12 Cookies

These crispy delicate cookies will please the whole family.

2 C. Finely Ground Almond Powder (Grind Almonds in Food Processor Until They Look Like Flour)
¼ Cup Xylitol
1 Tablespoons Almond Extract
1 Teaspoon Vanilla Extract
2 Eggs
1 Pinch salt
1 Tablespoons coconut Oil
½ Cup Pine Nuts (for garnish)

Preheat oven to 350 In a large bowl, mix well all ingredients except the pine nuts. Using a tablespoon or teaspoon (depending on what size cookie you want) scoop out a portion of the cookie batter, shape it into a ball, dip it in the pine nuts, and place on a cookie sheet that has been lined with waxed paper and rubbed with coconut or grapeseed oil. Bake for 12-20 minutes, depending on the size of the cookies, until the pine nuts start to brown. Allow to cool completely before removing from the pan, otherwise they will crumble apart.

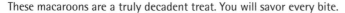

Chocolate Macaroons • Servings: 10-12 Cookies

These macaroons are a truly decadent treat. You will savor every bite.

Part 1 – Coconut Cookies
4-5 Egg Whites
1 Package of Unsweetened Shredded Coconut
2 Tablespoons. of Butter Melted.
Xylitol or Stevia to Sweeten

Beat egg whites until frothy. Stir in one package of unsweetened shredded coconut. Stir in melted butter. Add stevia or Xylitol to sweeten. Drop by teaspoon onto greased baking pan. Bake at 350° for 12 minutes. Cool in refrigerator until firm.

Part 2 – Chocolate Sauce
3 squares Unsweetened Chocolate
2 Tablespoons. of Coconut Oil
2 Tablespoons. of Butter
Xylitol or Stevia to Taste

Melt chocolate, coconut oil and butter together. Add Xylitol or stevia to sweeten. Dip coconut cookies in chocolate. Cool on wax paper. Keep refrigerated.

Lemon or Lime Ade • Servings: 1

Most lemonade is loaded with sugar, often even more than soda.
This is a much healthier way to enjoy lemonade.

2-3 Lemons or Limes
1 Cup Ice
2 Cups water

1 Teaspoon stevia or to Taste
Optional: 6-10 Whole Mint Leaves or to Taste

Juice lemons or limes into a blender or Vita-Mix®, add ice, water, stevia, and mint leaves if desired. Blend until frothy.

Authors

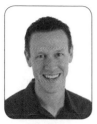

Dr. B.J. Hardick has consulted for natural healthcare clinics in the United States, Canada, and Europe for twenty years and is a co-founder of Maximized Living Canada. A highly sought-after speaker, and television and radio personality, Dr. Hardick has an active private practice in London, Ontario, where he maintains a special interest in nutrition, detoxification, children's health, and physical fitness.

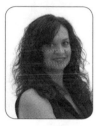

Kimberly Roberto manages one of America's leading wellness centers with her husband, Dr. Fred Roberto. Kimberly conducts popular cooking classes and exercise programs in person and online. She has led thousands of families to better health through personal-nutrition coaching. Kimberly and her husband reside outside Atlanta, Georgia, with their three children – James, Halle, and Ricky.

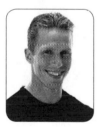

Dr. Ben Lerner is a *New York Times* best-selling author, U.S. Olympic Team doctor and World Team doctor, chairman of the USA Wrestling Wellness Advisory Council, chairman of Global Wellness for the Billion Soul Initiative, and co-founder of Maximized Living. Dr. Lerner lives in Celebration, Florida, with his wife, Dr. Sheri Lerner, and their three children – Skylar, Nicole, and Cael.